MAY
CAUSE
LOVE

MAY CAUSE LOVE

AN UNEXPECTED JOURNEY OF ENLIGHTENMENT AFTER ABORTION

KASSI UNDERWOOD

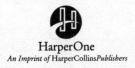

HarperOne
An Imprint of HarperCollinsPublishers

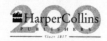

This is a work of nonfiction. The events and experiences detailed herein are all true and have been faithfully rendered as remembered by the author, to the best of her ability, or as told to the author by those who were present. Some names, physical descriptions and other identifying characteristics have been changed. The goal in all instances was to protect the privacy and anonymity of the individuals involved without damaging the integrity of the story.

FIRST EDITION

Designed by Yvonne Chan

Library of Congress Cataloging-in-Publication Data

Names: Underwood, Kassi, author.
Title: May cause love : an unexpected journey of enlightenment after abortion / Kassi Underwood.
Description: New York, NY : HarperOne, 2017. | Description based on print version record and CIP data provided by publisher; resource not viewed.
Identifiers: LCCN 2016043690 (print) | LCCN 2016030271 (ebook) | ISBN 9780062458650 (e-book) | ISBN 9780062458636 (hardback)
Subjects: LCSH: Underwood, Kassi. | Abortion—Psychological aspects. | Loss (Psychology) | Spiritual life. | Self-acceptance. | Self-realization. | BISAC: BIOGRAPHY & AUTOBIOGRAPHY / Personal Memoirs. | BIOGRAPHY & AUTOBIOGRAPHY / Women. | FAMILY & RELATIONSHIPS / Death, Grief, Bereavement.
Classification: LCC HQ767 (print) | LCC HQ767 .U53 2017 (ebook) | DDC 363.46—dc23
LC record available at https://lccn.loc.gov/2016043690

17 18 19 20 21 LSC(H) 10 9 8 7 6 5 4 3 2 1

For my mom

AUTHOR'S NOTE

This book is a blend of memoir and journalism and therefore a "true story," which means it is probably skewed by time lapses and unchecked emotions, but redeemed, I hope, by the due diligence of journals, interviews, conversations, research, and a good deal of self-examination. My friends and family in these pages generously granted me permission to share their stories, their letters, and sometimes their real names. My deepest thanks and gratitude to them all. I have changed some identifying details. There are no composite characters. I do my best to use language that includes all expressions of gender identity, except when the best available historical information and statistics refer only to women. I use exclusionary gendered language to depict eras of my life before I knew better.

There will be some who will understand.

—BUDDHA

CONTENTS

EMAIL TO MY NEW FRIEND FROM THE INTERNET

From: Courtney

To: Kassi

Date: July 9, at 10:28 pm EST

Subject: How can I get past this?

Hi Kassi,

   I'm a college freshman and had an abortion three weeks ago. I was Googling places to tell my story, and there aren't any. I read your newspaper article, which led me to your website. I don't have anyone else to talk to about it, mostly because I'm scared of what they will say. My mother had an abortion many years ago, but she doesn't understand why I'm struggling after mine. I'm always depressed, and there is nothing I can do to stop it. I don't regret my abortion, but I'm, like, what if I didn't have to do it? It's not religious guilt. I'm an atheist. I'm a strong person, but I feel like I'm not strong enough to get past this. You said you got through it. You became stronger. I want to know how.

From: Kassi

To: Courtney

Date: July 10, at 11:11 am EST

Subject: Re: How can I get past this?

Dear Courtney,

   I am so glad you emailed me.

In 2004, when I was nineteen years old and eight weeks pregnant, I searched the Internet for somebody who seemed reasonably normal and qualified to tell me that I could feel okay again after my abortion. I had read the statistic that approximately one in three American women will terminate a pregnancy in her lifetime, but I wasn't aware of a single person in my home state of Kentucky who ever had. When I searched the shelves of my college library for a memoir that might help, I found personal accounts of sex addiction, daddy issues, and scandalous European love affairs, but not abortion. So I get how trippy it is to be surrounded by a community that's both everywhere and nowhere. I remember brushing my teeth the night before my appointment, feeling nauseated and exhausted, thinking about the embryo gaining momentum inside of me, still wishing there was a woman I could talk to. I didn't find her, at least not back then, so I had to become her.

I talked about my abortion all the time. I told businessmen seated on the next barstool. Classmates, librarians, gas station attendants. I backpacked through Italy, Austria, Spain, and France and found people like you and me everywhere. I even kept in touch with my ex-boyfriend, the semi-father, though he and I lived thousands of miles apart by then.

On the third anniversary of my abortion, he sent me an email to let me know he had a girlfriend and that she was six months pregnant with their child. He named his daughter Jade, the same name I'd suggested for the baby he and I didn't have. Dressed in a pencil skirt and high heels, I walked to the office bathroom and collapsed in a heap on the floor. I thought, *F*ck. Him.* I thought, *I could have had the baby after all.* I thought, *Please quit crying and stand up before someone finds you here.*

I was twenty-two. I finally had what I thought it took to raise a child: A College Degree. A Handle on My Drinking. House Plants. My ex and his girlfriend had become pregnant in a situation that bore a striking resemblance to ours: they didn't have bachelor's degrees or sobriety or a home, but—this is what changed everything for me—they had the baby anyway.

So I had to ask myself the same question you asked me (perhaps rhetori-cally): what if I didn't have to terminate my pregnancy?

Over the next three years, I tried to ignore the question. I curled up in bed, eating canned salmon, rich in omega-3 fatty acids known to fight depression. My brain started attacking me. I thought about trying to med-itate. I blared *Access Hollywood* instead. On paper, I had the life I'd had in mind when I deferred motherhood—comfortable salary, fancy business card, cross-country moves, dates with weirdos—but it hadn't delivered on the promise of "fulfillment." The right side of my face bloomed with cystic acne, induced by secret rage. I routinely pulled over on the side of the road to double over with my head between my legs during spells of free-floating abortion panic. Nightmares of children invaded my sleep.

I told no one that I was suffering, even though I wasn't ashamed of my abortion. Lots of my friends had told me they'd terminated pregnancies in high school or college or even yesterday morning. I never hid mine, not for one day, but I did hide my thoughts and feelings about it.

Here was the good news: if I'd had a free choice about whether to keep my accidental pregnancy, then I also had the agency to create what I needed now. A road map for recovery.

I read personal essays by people in our "abortion club" and noticed a unifying theme: most writers included *A Disclaimer on My Status of Re-gret* and *A Final Word on Relief.* Everyone was either relieved or regretful. These two emotions did not appear together in one account, let alone in one person. It seemed like a conspiracy in which millions of women were bound to an implicit social contract to match their emotion to a political persuasion. "Pro-life" advocates argued that nobody should have a choice because some people wished they'd continued their pregnancies. There is no shame in regret. There's no shame in regretting an irreversible decision a person is forced to make during a time crunch imposed by the law and ramped up by one's own biology.

"Pro-choice" advocates quoted the old adage: "most women feel relieved." It's true. Some people don't have even a mild aftershock after a termination. Maybe your mother is one of them. But to feel relieved, by definition, means you have only "a *temporary* break in a generally tense or tedious situation." I relished my relief; it was exhilarating while it lasted.

I felt personally indebted to the warriors for reproductive justice. Because of them, I wasn't forced to give birth or to seek a back alley abortion. But the community I adored, in which I sought refuge and friendship, who I defended at cocktail parties in the Bible Belt, could not fully comprehend depression around abortion. A feminist priest laughed through her nose when I admitted I needed to heal. She sincerely thought I was joking. At a pro-choice panel, an activist suggested that the only people struggling after abortion were women who bought into religious shame. The audience broke into a spontaneous applause.

Depression feels like numbness, like nothingness, like your mind is not your own, but maybe a small part of why you're depressed is because you're onto something. The cultural lunacy around abortion is depressing.

But culture wasn't entirely to blame.

Life led me to the door of a tunnel after my abortion. Instead of facing down the dark, I sat at the opening and drank. I fell in lust with lots of guys on the wrong side of the tunnel. I meditated and traveled and got "super busy." Sometimes I said, "Tunnel? What tunnel?" Sometimes I psychoanalyzed: "This reminds me of a tunnel from childhood."

So how did I get through it?

My first step inside the tunnel was a step you've already taken. I said to myself, *I am depressed about my abortion.* Then I exchanged that clunker of a D-word for "sad." *I am sad.*

I decided that neither side in the political war had permission to tell my story for me. I had felt the prescribed liberation afterward, but I also had questions like you, and I didn't want to feel obligated to regret my decision or to pretend that my abortion was no more significant than the tonsillectomy I had in high school.

I sat on a meditation cushion and asked the universe to lead me to the healing forces. Sounds quaint, I know, but it worked. An answer came from a Buddhist teacher I admired who told me about a ritual to practice after abortion. Father Google introduced me to a whole world of women healers who had carved out such spaces all across the United States. So I set out on a road trip to meet this motley crew.

I leaned on a strong and steady self—a noble self much braver than me, yet part of me. You've got a self like that inside of you. She is the same strong self that emailed a random lady on the Internet, using words like "depression" and "abortion." The same self is asking, *What if I didn't have to do it?*

Today, I'm thirty-two, and I believe my ex-boyfriend's daughter, Jade, is an undercover saint. In Buddhism, there's a story to convey how unique each human being is: that the odds that I was born as me and that you were born as you are the same as that of a turtle in the ocean who pokes his head out of the water just once every hundred years, and the one time he emerges, he sticks his head into the middle of a inner tube. It's a strange comfort to think that Jade would not be here if I had continued my pregnancy. I'd wager that every baby born on this planet could not be here without the butterfly effect of somebody else's abortion.

But philosophy and chaos theory didn't stop me from questioning what had happened. I think healing begins when we ask questions with sucker-punch answers. *What if I didn't have to do it?* is a rough one. It's also worth answering with all the grit you've got. It's worth answering all sorts of serious questions about our abortions. In my case, the brutal truth is, I did not *have* to have my abortion. I could have had the baby. This realization made me feel so depressed at first that I was afraid I would never be the same again. And I haven't been. I am better. Jade saved me from a lifetime of familiar misery. I'm a happier person than before my abortion because I have tried to learn any lesson that jacked-up situation could teach me. I am afraid, but I keep asking the universe questions and paying attention to the answers, in whatever form they come. I once read that all healing is the relief of fear. So here's a question I like to ask myself: "What's the most healing thing I could do right now?"

You've already told me the answer: talk about your abortion, even though you are afraid. Talk about it *because* you're afraid. If it's too scary to tell the truth for yourself, then tell it for others and we'll all be free. Some people won't get it; that's okay. Just keep searching for the flicker in the distance. That's the rest of us—we're looking for your light, too.

I.
THE
FIRST
NOBLE
TRUTH

- 1 -

HELL

FIVE YEARS AFTERWARD — I woke up in my graduate housing apartment in Manhattan, squinting at a diagonal ray of sun. It streaked my face like one of those signs that crosses something out. My hair was stiff with sweat and matted to my forehead, my feverish cheek pressed into the damp pillow.

I was twenty-four and had spent five years chasing my dreams like someone was holding a gun to my head. Here I was, eight stories above the honking taxicabs, a student at Columbia University, working to make my abortion a worthwhile investment, trying to become happy.

Last night seemed promising: the guy I thought I would marry came through the city on business and asked me out to dinner. I met him at the restaurant in tall black boots and dangly gold earrings, ready to strike a match and reignite the romance I had decimated. Halfway through the meal, he told me he was settling down with someone else.

And I woke up the next morning with the universe crossing me out.

Life is suffering. It's the First Noble Truth of Buddhism. (And one of the only things I knew about Buddhism.) But couldn't I at least suffer better?

This is a question that beckoned me to move forward, and then it stretched me back.

———————

ALL THE WAY BACK TO MY second year on the planet. To a hospital room in Lexington, Kentucky. Spindly and quiet, I sat on a chair in a cotton eyelet dress, clutching my newborn brother. He gazed up at me with marine blue eyes that matched our father's. I wanted to jump off the chair in my black patent leather shoes and make a run for it with Rusty in my arms, but my mother watched us from the bed, her gown bunched up around her shoulders. Dad lifted my brother out of my arms and replaced him with a new doll. With her corn-silk ringlets and blue-green eyes, she could have passed for a third sibling, but she was cold and stiff, smelled like rubber.

Over the next decade, I memorized the path to motherhood—each step in my parents' story. You met in high school. You got engaged at twenty-four. You sashayed down the aisle in a white lace gown with a twenty-foot train. You lived in a classic redbrick colonial and twirled the night away on the dance floor, then gathered in the pews of an old church the next morning. I had come to earth the day before their fourth wedding anniversary. The way I understood it, you didn't just wait until marriage to have children. You waited for marriage, then four more years.

According to family lore, my parents fell in love because their fathers were political enemies. My mother was a Southern Baptist Republican sorority sister who enjoyed filet mignon and earned a master's degree in education. My father sported a green military field jacket as an F-you to the establishment, ate a diet that excluded red meat, dropped out of college and never went back. Soon after my parents' courtship began, Dad attempted to fit a traditional mold. He cut off his brown John Lennon shag, traded his buffalo sandals for the "Lexington tuxedo"—collared shirt, khaki pants, and penny loafers sans socks—and started a homebuilding business.

THE FIRST EIGHT YEARS OF MY life were ridiculously charmed. Balancing a video camera on his shoulder, my dad filmed three-year-old me jogging laps around our backyard fence and hollered, "Good job, Kassi Moto!" I pretended not to hear him cheering, but in a letter I mailed later to a local news station, I declared that he deserved a crown on his head for being the best dad in the world. The Fox 56 Kids' Club named him the Father of the Year.

Nana, my mother's mom, had me beat for the title of his Biggest Fan.

She would pull up in her blue Mercedes convertible with a floral scarf wrapped around her head. "Knock-knock," she'd sing, letting herself in, dresses with price tags piled over her arm, a new brass lamp in one hand, and a glossy furniture catalogue in the other. "I've got goodies."

"Mom, you shouldn't have," my mother said with a southern drawl. She stood five foot three, same height as my grandmother. She was a middle child, the second youngest of four, a birth order that gave her an invisibility complex. Mom resembled Heather Locklear from *Melrose Place*, but she thought she was as eye-catching as a slice of Wonder Bread. Her parents were broke until she started undergrad, when her father's business finally brought windfall. Nana planned her wedding and her career, filled her closet with designer dresses, and furnished our home with a fancy piano. I thought Nana was the town mayor, tottering along the sidewalk in kitten heels, firing off orders with her good-natured drawl. *The stop sign would really pop in turquoise.* All eight grandchildren worshipped Nana, though she made me feel like I was the only one.

"Kass, show Nana what a good big sister you are," my mother said. Scrambling up on the couch, I supported Rusty's bobble-head with one hand and his bum with the other, beaming up at my mother, father, and grandmother while they snapped Polaroid photos and patted my head.

"She's a natural with children," Nana said. I pictured her fairy wand tapping me on the forehead and waited for further instruction to turn out like her. The foundational principles of the domestic goddess included wearing monochromatic getups to slenderize your figure, taking short steps like a sandpiper, and pulling the crotch of your swimsuit to the side in the restroom instead of taking it off—you didn't want to take too long and give people the wrong impression.

"Wouldn't your daddy look handsome in this tuxedo?" Nana asked me.

"Very," I said, reaching up to touch the smooth sleeve of the suit. My father—he was lanky with dark curls—laughed bashfully, seeming unaccustomed to receiving such lavish praise.

"Wouldn't your mama be the belle in this?" Nana said, turning the hanger to display a green dress with sequins that looked like scales on a mermaid's tail. I nodded. What a dress!

ONE MORNING, WHEN I WAS EIGHT and my mother was thirty-six, we knocked on Nana's front door and she answered it completely baldheaded from chemotherapy. I thought the breast cancer treatments would work and her hair would grow back, but we buried her a month later. My grandfather remarried within the year.

A black scrim fell over all of us. My father studied a newspaper called the *Daily Racing Form* at the kitchen table with a tumbler of vodka and a blank expression I didn't recognize. Rusty came home from the elementary school playground with two black eyes. Mom ground out a seventy-hour workweek, teaching public school English. I quit horseback riding since Nana wasn't alive to cart me to lessons and took up smoking cigarettes with a friend, crouching down in a drainage pipe in a nearby park.

Over the years after Nana died, faucets stayed broken. Doors became loose on the hinges. There was one room in our house that nobody lived in; a portrait of my grandmother, decked out in a mink coat, hung on its wall. Nana had decorated the room with her extravagant touch, furnishing it with a piano and a camelback sofa. Sometimes, when I traipsed down the steps, I caught my mother standing alone in the room, staring at the portrait with her arms crossed.

I missed my grandmother terribly, but it didn't occur to me that my mother was sad because her mother was dead. I didn't know what grief looked like or how ungrieved grief could pile up on the psyche like debts. I thought I was restless and uncomfortable because the vibe at home felt like trying to breathe with a plastic bag over my head. I knew I wanted to get out of Kentucky, and if I had to stay in Kentucky, then I at least wanted to get out of the house.

The opposite happened. I was often grounded for mouthing off. When I told my mother I felt uncomfortable with the hierarchy between parents and children, she grounded me longer for questioning her authority. In an effort to parlay my love of kids into financial freedom, I started babysitting in sixth grade, but I couldn't bring myself to enforce rules upon the pint-sized humans. Instead, we built couch-cushion forts and stayed up past bedtime, eating cereal out of the box, and marching through the halls, banging pots and pans with spoons. I took myself on shopping sprees at the mall with the crumpled-up dollar bills of my independence, but even in a new tube top, freedom seemed as elusive as the state line.

When I was thirteen, a friend of mine plunked an amber bottle of whiskey on a lowboy in her bedroom with white lace frills around the windows. I guzzled it back without chaser. The whiskey burned my veins until I went numb and floated around her family's old southern mansion on a pink cumulous cloud, fortified with the kind of divine love that gives you inner peace and courage. It was five minutes of nirvana. Then a blackout, during which I vaguely recall crawling up a staircase on all fours. The next year, dressed in high heels, I snuck airplane bottles of wine into my purse and smoked menthols at a deli near my high school and fantasized about falling in love.

I wasn't a star in the classroom. I bagged a few literary awards but nearly flunked out. I got suspended for having a smoke in the locker room while the other girls ran drills in gym. I was grounded for weeks after failing tests or missing midnight curfew. Dad marked his vodka bottle with a Sharpie pen each evening to keep me from stealing his booze.

In occasional efforts to feel good alone and au naturel, I read Buddhist wisdom and *Life's Little Instruction Book* and became a good Christian and tried yoga. I searched for a magic and a mindset that would make sense to me, the way Star Wars and Harry Potter made sense to my friends. Motherhood would be my religion, I thought, the one good thing I'd do. A family of my own represented freedom to me, liberation from the rules of home and the power to govern myself. I figured I'd better con some sucker into marrying me first.

BY AGE FOURTEEN, I MOISTURIZED MY neck three times a day to preserve my youthful appearance well into marriage. My monthly subscription of *Elle Décor* was dog-eared with home furnishing ideas. I wanted ten kids and kept a running list of baby names. I put on a ruffled apron and served up grilled cheese sandwiches to my stoned guy friends, who'd sit at my mother's kitchen table where I could listen and take mental notes. I may have rebelled against my parents, but I conformed to any law a teenage boy offhandedly laid down. If I'd spent half the time on my schoolwork as on preparations for domestic bliss, Mama said, I might have been a candidate for Harvard, but I wanted to be a candidate for a boy's last name. I saw myself as the maternal type, the kind who could stay Zen like Marge, fold pants like Martha, bake like Julia, drink like Dorothy. Didn't matter that half those ladies weren't even parents. By my Virgin Mary logic, building a strong marriageability quotient meant abstaining from the version of sex that causes pregnancy until after the wedding.

I had never seen a gynecologist. I had never seen a pregnant teenager. None of my friends had sex, as far as I knew. I was under the impression that no one I knew had been born out of wedlock. Health class followed the lead of George W. Bush. In my four years of high school, the Bush Administration allocated 302 million federal dollars to an education that encouraged teenagers to abstain from sex until marriage, using tactics like passing an unwrapped York Peppermint Pattie around the room to show how "dirty" a girl becomes after being held in so many hands.

I somehow thought Planned Parenthood was a conservative Christian organization and was pretty sure abortion was illegal. Otherwise, I reasoned, my cousins wouldn't be permitted to protest in front of clinics and block women from entering them. I didn't know anybody who'd admittedly terminated a pregnancy. I had no idea that upward of fifty million abortions occurred worldwide each year, that approximately one in three American women would have one by age forty-five.

Billboards with antiabortion messages studded the highways, giving me the impression that a woman lost her mind after an abortion and never got it back again. At school lunch, a classmate relayed her Christian preacher's message about the wayward mothers who murdered their babies. This mythical creature-woman was considered a mentally ill whore, a moral outlaw. Just thinking about her, I felt eons away from God. I thought terminating was the worst thing that could possibly happen to a human being, the worst thing anybody could do.

Pushing fifteen, in retro winged eyeliner like Brigitte Bardot, I crouched behind the sheer white drapes of my bedroom window. I wore bellbottoms and blue platform heels. I ashed my cigarette on the sill, scribbling the names of my imaginary children in a notebook: *Jade,* I wrote, and then set it on the nubby brown carpet and pushed it under the bed.

I modeled my ideal future on my best friend Charlie's family: her parents raised a brood of six on a panoramic green horse farm. All the kids were tall and fair-skinned and freckled and hilarious. Charlie and I would recruit one of them to come with us down a winding black road until we reached the horses. There, they'd film the music videos we'd choreographed. Sporting all-white costumes with rainbow wigs, we'd lip-synch to the *Reality Bites* and *Jackie Brown* soundtracks while skipping back and forth in front of the plank fence, swinging our arms in slow motion with somber frowns. I had so much fun it felt illegal. Every time I thought her mom was coming outside to tell us we were in trouble, it would turn out she was just bringing us a snack or a prop she thought would improve the video. Still dressed in our costumes, we'd sit down for dinner at Charlie's kitchen table. It was so big the dishes had to be passed around on a revolving tray. I wanted my own giant family on a lolling horse farm. I'd sport cowgirl boots and green sequins with a glamorous 'do like Dolly Parton and fuel up the team on beans and vegetables. (I had quit eating meat, like my dad.) My husband would be tall and fine, steady and trustworthy, and madly in love with me.

TRAIPSING DOWN THE SIDEWALK IN CUTOFFS and spaghetti straps, almost fifteen years old, I heard the honk of a car horn—Kentucky's catcall. I was about to flip off the driver when I heard him yell my name. Actually, he said, "Mama Kass!"

Like the lead singer of The Mamas & the Papas.

I turned back and his face came into view: flipped-up black lashes, a sun-streaked mess of dark hair, pronounced cheekbones, framed in

the driver's window of a boxy red Isuzu Trooper. I had seen him earlier, standing on the other side of the pool. He was summer-browned
and lanky. Drenched khaki shorts hung off his hips. They were a tad
short. I'd thought, if it's possible to fall in love at first sight, then I
just did.

He spun a U-turn over the curb and cruised up next to me, stub-
bing a cigarette butt in the car ashtray. His eyes slammed into mine.

"Hay," he said. His name was Will-B VanMeter. "Want a ride?"

His voice was deep and gravely, lazy-sounding, slightly lispy, but
articulate, with an inflection so contagious I thought he'd invented
the local vernacular. *Hay,* he said, the way you'd call a horse. *Hay,*
we'd all say. I liked the grammar of his name, Will Be, the future progressive tense, *an ongoing continuous action that would be occurring in the
future,* but it was glaringly deficient in a verb. We Will-B doing what?

The passenger door swung open. Two bare feet slapped down on the
blacktop. It was another boy, Barrett, in red swim trunks. He presented
the shotgun seat with a flourish of the hands. I hoisted myself onto
the cloth seat. A green Celtics shirt clung to Will-B's concave chest. He
wasn't a Celtics fan. I firmly doubted he'd ever been to Boston.

I let Will-B light my cigarette at a stoplight. It was the end of June,
his sixteenth birthday. He had picked up his learner's permit a few
hours earlier and stole off in Barrett's brother's stick shift. He parked
behind his mother's green Volkswagen that had a bumper sticker
plastered on it protesting the new houses my father built: *Growth De-
stroys the Bluegrass Forever.* Our parents were political enemies, just like
my grandparents. Will-B's father had a famous horse farm. I wanted
to be a housewife on a horse farm.

It was all coming together.

His mother walked out on the covered front porch of her little
pink house. I flicked my cigarette into the street. Will-B stuck his
cigarette in his mouth like a wheat head and gave his mother a hug.

They were on a first-name basis. She wasn't a curls-and-pearls country club mom. She looked like she'd stepped out of a 1970s album cover, dressed like me in a bohemian shirt with her long, dark hair parted down the middle. We shared the same birthday in August, an astrological coincidence I suspected was a sign from God. Will-B lived alone with her, though he had two older brothers in their twenties and two younger siblings who lived with his father and stepmother. When Barrett and his mother went inside, Will-B and I sat on the warm concrete front steps. He pivoted in his seat and said, "Will you go out with me?"

Translation: will you be my girlfriend?

"Yes," I replied.

We locked eyes for a solid minute while the end of his cigarette turned to ash.

All summer, he hoofed it on foot back and forth the two miles between our parents' homes. We sat in my tree house with his buddies, pecking at warm beer cans until my midnight curfew. When his crew filed out the back fence, he lagged behind and laid a wet one on me. It wasn't my first kiss, but it sure felt like it. With him, I could see where a kiss could lead. I was in the market for a longer session, preferably without his friends around, but I couldn't get him alone. Each night, I'd have to wait for his posse to get scarce before he'd make a move.

Near September, Will-B snuck into my backyard by himself. We scaled the ladder to my tree house and sat with our bare legs touching. After two hours of holding hands and sharing a Camel with me, he finally leaned toward me to make a play.

My dog started barking at the back storm door. My mother burst out on the steps in a cotton nightgown, drawling at Will-B to get gone. I hopped to the ground.

"Inside, Kass," she snapped.

"Mama, no. Please," I yelled, running to her across the lawn with my hands in the air. Will-B darted toward the back gate and let himself out with a clank. "Will-B, don't go. Mama! Why are you doing this to me?"

"You're making out with a boy in the backyard. He didn't even give you a fifteenth birthday present," she said matter-of-factly as she grabbed my hand and pulled me over the threshold of the house, the noise of the television and my father snoring on the couch in his bathrobe.

"I don't need a birthday present," I shrieked, tossing myself on the floor.

"Have some respect for yourself. If he's interested, he'll care enough to give you a present."

"He says it's in the mail," I told her.

"Gimme a break, Kass." She shook her head.

A week later, Will-B called me from his father's farm. "We need to talk," he said. I was in bed sniffling pitifully, but I was not a fool—I had my break-up speech prepared. Mom was standing in the doorway of my bedroom when I hung up the phone.

"The present wasn't in the mail, was it," she said.

"No," I replied, holding my gaze on the top of my homemade fishnet canopy.

Will-B switched to my school in the fall, our sophomore year, and started dating an experienced senior who I was sure gave him more than I had. I dated a senior of my own, then Will-B and I both became single again. The rest of high school, we kissed in backseats, garages, on the couch in the pink house, but he never tried anything more advanced than a three-hour make-out session. I could wake up with him and with every stitch of clothing intact.

I never told my hometown girlfriends about my feelings for him. I wasn't the least bit private, especially about my infatuations, but I felt that our connection was spiritual, sanctified from above. When I had the blues, my father would knock on my bedroom door and say, "Will-B's on the phone, Moto." Talking to him reminded my teenage brain that I wouldn't be trapped at home forever—I could end up on a farm with him and six kids. I scribbled in my journal that he was the spiritual practice I'd sought in Buddhist wisdom, yoga, and agape, even in motherhood itself. Something holy was happening here.

Senior year, we shared a biology textbook as an excuse to see each other under the auspices of homework. On a stopover at the pink house where we had arranged for the latest textbook exchange, Will-B's mother answered the door and told me he'd asked her to send me to his bedroom. I stamped up the creaking wooden steps in t-strap platforms. I had been fourteen when we had met, was now seventeen, had distracted myself with other relationships, but my feelings for him grew back like fingernails.

His room was monkishly clean and quiet. He was lying supine on the far side of the bed with the textbook in his lap. We stared at each other for an awkward beat. I wanted to snatch the biology book from his hand and throw it against the wall and start the transcendent love affair I'd imagined when I'd seen him on the other side of the deep end three years earlier. Break my Virgin Mary rule. Marry him and have his children and race lawn mowers in the summer. Flustered, I crawled across the bed on my hands and knees, tore the hardback from his stubborn grip, and wiggled backwards until I stood to my feet.

When prom came along, he took another girl.

Heartbroken, I closed my eyes and threw a dart at a map. Then I left the bourbon barrels and tobacco fields, the bouncy bluegrass fiddle, the long tar roads and black plank fences, miles and miles of red river, the scalped mountains in Appalachia, and the Ten Commandments mounted on public property. I left the town where I grew up, with its southern manners and pierced anarchists in vegan leather vests, its midnight screening of *The Rocky Horror Picture Show* and national reputation as a gay haven, where the antiabortion billboards seemed as natural as the dogwood trees. I applied blindly to a college I had never visited, in a state I had never stepped foot in, in a town as far away from home as my parents would permit me to run.

I LOVED VERMONT. "THE UNIVERSITY OF VERMIN," my father said. Jagged mountaintops, green license plates. Being nicknamed "Kentucky." Dabbling in drugs without getting grounded.

One morning, I'd curled up in bed, reeling from an overindulgence of speed and weed, plus an eighth of psychedelic mushrooms, sincerely afraid that I was about to die. I blinked at the dorm phone on the wall, debating whether to call my parents and say goodbye.

The phone started to ring.

It was Will-B, calling to see if I was okay, at 4 A.M. on Monday.

I was the token virgin among my northeastern college friends. I assumed their birth control pills and condoms had worked, because none of them had children. But the only guy I'd wanted to break my virginity mission for—Will-B—hadn't seemed to want it.

Determined to let him go, I started dating a Jewish philosophy major with a halo of curls. A week in, I obtained a rectangular package of birth control pills, which I punched out of tinfoil and swallowed at the same millisecond each morning. With hormones, a Trojan, and a pull-out plan, I was triple-protected, eighteen years old. After finally losing my virginity, my predominant thought was, *a long run for a short slide.*

Extremely sexy side effects of the birth control pill included bloating, a short fuse in reaction to inanimate objects (like snowflakes landing on my nose), and existential terror about the meaninglessness of basketball. I stood at my window, watching the boys shoot hoops on the court below, wondering, *What's the point? The game will only end.*

I liked the philosophy major, but when he suggested that I lose both my Freshman 30 and my downhome accent, I wished him well and let my birth control lapse. Getting laid wasn't worth the trouble of Ortho Tri-Cyclen and the antidepressant Effexor XR, to prevent pregnancy. The point of waiting until marriage was to avoid getting knocked up by somebody who didn't want to marry me, so I gave my moral code a tweak: no sex until engagement.

Will-B dropped out of college and enlisted in the army. I could have sworn he was a peace-loving hippie like my father, what with his undisciplined hair, passive disposition, and Rusted Root blaring out the windows of his car. I'd never even known him to play a sport. Over the phone, he told me he idolized his war vet grandfather and was caught up in the patriotic fever after 9-11, the romance of a young man going off to combat and fighting for his country.

His cousin Hock dropped him off at the recruitment station in Lexington. There, his long malt locks were shaved off, a necklace was strung around his neck with a silver dog tag. Then, with a team of other recruits, he was put on a plane to Fort Sill, Oklahoma, for basic training.

He tore up the phone lines calling me on Sundays while I puttered around my dorm room. We sent letters back and forth. When the semester was over, I went back to Lexington for the summer.

Riding out to a field party in Bourbon County, Will-B and I chatted casually while I studied his military look. Thousands of pushups had sculpted his skinny arms into marble. He had a new haircut, a faux hawk that accentuated his long black lashes and dense brows.

Coincidentally, we'd booked flights out of Lexington on the same date, scheduled three weeks away. Mine would go to California, his to South Korea for a yearlong tour in the DMZ.

"What's the DMZ, exactly?" I asked.

"The Demilitarized Zone," he said. "What's in California?"

"A road trip. Arnold Schwarzenegger. Avocados."

At the field party—which is Kentucky shorthand for a keg party on a farm with cars parked around a bonfire—we sat on the bed of his SUV with the back gate open. Legs dangling, sipping bitter beer foam from red cups and watching the flames. After all the phone calls and letters, we had come to an understanding that we were together now. He squeezed my leg and told me he wanted to be committed, stay true to each other during his year away.

I felt an intoxicating rush of joy. Finally. Finally. But we'd be separated longer than the time it takes to make a baby.

"It's only a year," Will-B said. It sounded like a decade, an eternity.

Too soon, we were parting again. He suited up in olive fatigues with a sharp-shouldered camouflage coat. His tan combat boots clomped against the hardwood floor. He handed me a soft gray fleece embroidered with the crest of his father's farm. I held the fleece to my nose and we boarded separate flights to our alliterative destinations, Korea and California. We still hadn't had sex.

BACK IN VERMONT, I BECAME THE dorm expert on the politics of Kim Jong-il. My room smelled like a funeral home from all the flowers he sent. I shopped plane tickets to Korea and installed a webcam with a flat black eye above my computer. Pixilating on the screen, he looked strapping in button-down shirts I embroidered with his initials and sent flying to his eastern barracks. Wearing overalls and a long tawny braid down her back, my roommate, Ruby, thought our "webcam time," as she called it, was hilariously creepy. It was 2003, before Skype and FaceTime.

Over the phone, eleven thousand miles away, Will-B told me he loved me. I wanted more. I wanted him to say he always had. I wanted him to explain why he'd waited until he was moving halfway around the planet to start a relationship. He didn't.

We communicated constantly, over oceans, through time zones. I tacked a photograph of his newborn niece over my desk, taped a picture of us on the cement wall next to my bunk: he's kissing me the devastating way a soldier kisses a loyal girl before he ships off. I'm kissing him back like I am that girl—but a seed of resentment grew day by day.

One night, there was a knock at the door. I was sitting at my dorm desk, immersed in conversation with Will-B over the computer. I overheard Ruby talking in the animated shorthand of old friends. Will-B had to scoot off to breakfast—it was dinner in my time zone—so I said bye to the square of light and closed my laptop with a click. I introduced myself to the guy in the doorway.

"Noah," he said. His hand felt warm and dangerous, like a gun.

I'd recently devoured Erica Jong's *Fear of Flying*, a novel that sold twenty million copies and introduced to my vocabulary the "zipless f*ck." The zipless f*ck "is free of ulterior motives," involves "no talk at *all*." In the "ultimate zipless A-1 f*ck," "you never get to know the man very well." I was impressed with the boldness of it, the carelessness and the freedom of sex without further solicitations.

"Zipless," Jong writes, "because when you came together zippers fell away like rose petals, underwear blew off in one breath like dandelion fluff."

Noah took off his hat. His Grateful Dead jacket shifted over his back while he crossed the room and eased into a chair by the window. Ruby and I sat on the floral couch across from him. Noah seemed eccentric and cagey in a Joaquin Phoenix sort of way, but he looked like River Phoenix. Feminine beauty and hair, hair, hair. He was twenty, had a soft-spoken hoarse voice. He'd just traveled seventeen hours from a concert in my hometown, of all places. I took three icy beer cans from the mini fridge and passed one to Ruby and another to Noah.

"I'm on probation, actually," he said.

"Noah's always up to no good," Ruby said, shaking her head. Noah said he intended to earn a bachelor's degree, stay clean this time. He was a ski lift operator, just enrolled in community college. He'd rented a room on the north end of Burlington.

He left his hat on the dresser that night and stopped by to pick it up after I got off work. My place of employment was Glad Rags, a vintage shop where I repaired dresses in a small sewing room behind a red velvet curtain. Noah told me he was heading to Olive Garden for dinner and invited me to come along. I said yes because I was a sucker for that bottomless salad.

I expected him to act like a brooding young convict, but he surprised me with a Slapstick Dad sense of humor, tucking his napkin in his shirt at the restaurant. Later, back in the dorm, he put on Ruby's floppy hat and joke-seductively danced, pulling up his T-shirt with one finger. I laughed until I clambered up to my bunk bed, in a wasted blur, knocking the snapshot of Will-B and me loose as I pulled the down comforter up to my neck. Noah followed up behind me. After putting back a beer, he couldn't risk driving home while on probation—he hadn't hit the legal drinking age. I flipped over and straightened out the crooked photograph, leaving a foot between Noah and me. Nothing happened.

Nothing was going to happen.

Will-B called me from night watch in his Humvee in the valley of the silver rock mountains of Korea. I was sipping vodka from a Nalgene bottle, ensconced in a cubby at the library, doodling my married name in a notebook: Kassi VanMeter. He told me I was the last person he thought about at night and the first person he thought about in the morning.

Later, Ruby and I were hosting our regular event, an evening of drinking and dancing in which all who gathered pounded a shot of box wine per minute, cued by a mix CD with songs lasting sixty seconds. Friends packed the room, including Noah. Full of shots, I danced dizzily into the hallway, toward the bathroom, when suddenly, stupidly, I was kissing Noah in the stairwell. Then in his truck. Then in his quiet bedroom on the north end. He was my second sex, after the philosophy major.

I woke up hungover and in disbelief that I had done this behind Will-B's back. Afraid that I'd end up alone, I decided to make Noah my boyfriend, too. Over the next week, he twirled me across the sloping floors of his ramshackle apartment while I gripped a vodka bottle. I swung back and forth between trying to fit us into the zipless f*ck category and trying to make it a real relationship.

"I love you," I slurred, thinking I had to love him now.

"You're confused," Noah said. He and I collapsed on his ratty couch after dancing. He leaned over the coffee table, crushing up OxyContin—hillbilly heroin—and snorting the powder through a rolled-up dollar bill. He swore to me that he never shot up, but his stovetop collection of spoons were all bent, their silver charred to black.

After he had passed his last urine test with his probation officer, he opened a dresser drawer in his bedroom and revealed to me his actual rap sheet: a manila folder bound by green rubber bands, thick as a study Bible. Instead of church clothes, he had "court clothes."

Two weeks later, Noah dropped out of school. His suburban parents, unhappy with his performance—he'd already been kicked out of his first college—drove up from Massachusetts and confiscated his pickup truck until he cleaned up his act. Without transportation to work, he lost his gig at the ski lift and started paying rent by selling OxyContin to a fat man in a minivan whose children watched from car seats as he passed wads of cash through the window. I waited on the sidewalk, sipping vodka from a Diet Coke can. We had sex every day for a month.

Given my bad reaction to the birth control pill, I decided to forgo hormonal contraception and dragged Noah along with me to see a doctor about an IUD that would sit in my uterus like a T-shaped bouncer. Much to my surprise, the doctor said no. She judged the relationship as "too new" for an IUD, implying that, in the event that Noah infected me with an STD, I'd be rendered infertile when I wanted to have children. She assured us that condoms were a perfectly effective way to prevent pregnancy without hormones. Part of me wanted to insist that she give me an IUD—my brother and I both were products of birth control failures—but I didn't want to jeopardize my chance to become a mother, and her professional opinion made me think that my triple method of birth control had been a neurotic hangover from the Bible Belt. Condoms were all that Noah and I used, but we used them religiously.

On Saint Patrick's Day, I stayed late in my underwear design course, sewing bones to a corset. Scraps of fabric were strewn along the draper's table where I worked. Clad in a threadbare flannel shirt, Noah had stopped in to help me clip the bones. My period was late.

"If it hasn't come by April, we'll take the test," he whispered.

ON THE FIRST OF APRIL, I was limping down a hospital hallway clutching my medical records to my chest for a different test. My foot was inexplicably swollen and painful. I passed stretchers and wheelchairs and searched for the x-ray room. A freezing cold wind rattled the windows. I had a heightened sense of smell and felt nauseated from the blended odors of rubbing alcohol and musky skin. My period hadn't started yet.

Please, I prayed. *Lord, I'd rather die than be pregnant.*

I was nineteen.

Seated on the exam table, I let my boot hit the floor, and pulled off my wool sock. The ponytailed x-ray technician grabbed a white machine that hung down from the ceiling and positioned it next to my foot. Her hair was pulled back so tightly that it raised her eyebrows, giving her a look of perpetual disbelief.

"Any chance you could be pregnant?" she asked. "Radiation can harm a baby," she added.

This was a unique burden of womanhood: seeing the doctor for a foot injury resulted in my confessing my recent sexual adventures to three strangers.

"My period's a little late," I said to the x-ray tech. "But I probably miscalculated the date."

The tech and her two male assistants grabbed heavy lead smocks from a hook on the wall and draped them over my shoulders and back. The room went black, then flickered.

In an exam room, the doctor, a small olive-skinned man with brown puddles for eyes, thumbed the x-ray.

"Foot fracture," he said. He modulated his speech like a shrink. "Nothing you can do but try not to walk until you mend."

I sat up at the edge of the exam table and zipped into my retro blue ski coat. And then blurted out, "Do y'all do pregnancy tests?"

The doctor glanced up from a chart.

"Yes. Give me a minute," he replied, stepping out the door.

A nurse in a long white lab coat led me to a bathroom with stainless steel plating every surface. I peed into a small sample container, tightened the lid, and slid it back through the window to the laboratory. I sat in the front row of the waiting room and clasped my hands in my lap. My first pregnancy was supposed to be about joy. I was supposed to call my mother and make her guess what. I was supposed to be married four years. I was supposed to be twenty-eight. That first positive pregnancy test was supposed to mark the beginning of my life.

- 2 -

THE END OF APRIL

The lab door at the university clinic swung open and out walked a nurse in a crisp white coat. I studied her face for a preview of the results, expecting eye contact, a look of reassurance, but she merely sailed past me with a manila envelope. Her heels pumped the carpet.

The doctor appeared, wearing a strange smile, and beckoned me. I followed him down the hall, focused on the rigid collar of his shirt.

The room we wordlessly entered was not an exam room, but his personal office. He crossed his legs and folded his hands around one knee. When he bowed his head, I knew.

"F*ck," I said to him, myself, everyone, everything.

I rocked back and forth in the chair, muttering all variations of *f*ck*.

"That's why there are options," said the doctor.

"I would never do that," I shot back.

That he took me for the kind of girl who'd get rid of it nearly startled my tears dry.

Noah called me half a minute later, when I was still in the chair at the doctor's desk. My ringer was set to the William Tell Overture, which reminded me of *The Lone Ranger,* which reminded me of horses, which reminded me of Will-B, which reminded me that everything was ruined. I hadn't even had sex with the guy I loved, but here I was pregnant with a guy I hardly knew. This was not the plan.

"Noah?" I sniveled into my flip phone. "The test was positive."

"Oh, f*ck," he said. He would be here in two minutes.

My fragmented thoughts began to fuse into whole questions, the first of which was to wonder whether there was another exit.

"I can't walk back through that waiting room," I told the doctor. I was sure that everyone in the waiting room was onto me. They'd seen the nurse take me to the bathroom, noticed the doctor's somber disposition when he called me back into his office.

"Don't worry," he replied. "Patients bawl over mono."

NOAH DROVE ME TO GLAD RAGS and parked out front.

I sucked in a deep breath and flipped the mirror. Eyeliner had streaked down my cheeks, looking more warrior paint than Bardot *Je Joue.*

I left Noah in the car. The mannequins in the store window wore shiny prom getups, top hats and blue boas, pastel gowns pinched at the waist. Inside, Johnny Cash crooned prison lore through the speakers hanging above the row of fringed cowgirl skirts. The store smelled mustier than usual, like dust and old woman perfume.

Dez, my boss, was sorting wigs. Seeing my smeared eye makeup, she stopped and beckoned me toward the staircase leading down to the basement. I felt burglarized, only the thief was still in this house, sheltered by me. I followed Dez's black pixie haircut down creaking steps to her "office," a desk hemmed in by racks of polyester pants and 1960s circle capes.

"I'm pregnant," I cried. I expected her to gasp and hug me, but instead she walked off into the tunnels of polyester and dragged out a red high-heel chair, the kind sold in novelty stores. I collapsed into it.

"With perfect use, condoms are only 98 percent effective," Dez said. "We're all statistics. You know what you gotta do."

I was only nineteen, but I felt so old.

"It's selfish," I said. "No offense."

For all my dithering, it couldn't be denied that the first person I sought out after I found out I was pregnant was also the only person I knew who'd had an abortion.

Dez started ticking off the reasons why it would be more selfish to have a child—a list I admit was abridged: "You're a teenager. You drink like a washed-up child actor. Noah sells drugs—"

"He—"

"Don't. I know everybody in this town." She lit a cigarette, shook the match. "I've run with guys like him all my life. Rehab's next. Jail. Doubt he'll make it to thirty-five. Don't be selfish, doll. Don't have a child to spare your own guilt. End it and live with it like the rest of us."

"Don't you regret it?"

"Regret being irresponsible? You bet. Any time you have sex, you could get pregnant. Sex and babies. Make the connection." She knocked my head with a loose fist and flipped through the Yellow Pages in her lap. "Kass, it's no bigger than a fingernail."

That helped. A little. A fingernail was not a life in a liminal stage.

"What does it feel like?" I asked.

"The worst cramps you've ever had."

"But I don't get cramps."

"Don't tell your mother about this," Dez added.

"I tell my mother everything."

"Not this," she replied, clenching a cigarette with her teeth. "You'll break her heart."

She took the phone off the wall and handed it to me. She dialed Planned Parenthood and let me listen to the recording about my three options: "Keep the pregnancy and keep the baby, keep the pregnancy and give up the child for adoption, or abortion. Choose what is best for you."

None of the options were appealing.

When I hung up the phone, Dez slapped my knee. "Why don't you take a break from work for a while, Party Girl?"

I needed a vacation. And she needed to fire me.

I PACED THE NARROW PATH BETWEEN my bed and the wall of dead musicians, a thousand miles from my childhood bedroom.

"Mom?" I held the phone to my ear with both hands.

"What's wrong baby?" she asked. Shame clawed at my throat, altered my voice.

"Nothing, Mama. It's—" But I detonated. I tried to muster "nothing at all," but it came out more like *Natal. It's natal.*

I heard my father in the background. "She's pregnant, isn't she?"

It was our collective worst nightmare.

"Are you?" my mother asked.

". . ."

"Oh, Kassi," she said. It was a whisper like a bellow.

I apologized and inhaled with a stutter.

"Whatever decision you make will be a terrible one for you," she said, "But if you keep the baby, come on home. We'll raise the child here."

I heard: *if you keep the baby, moving back home is your only option.* As soon as she said those words, I realized what they meant. *Raise,* she said, a whine of a verb: eighteen years yawning out into my future, the worry, the laundry. *The child,* she said, meaning the heart bulge inside my body. *Here,* she said, always looking for a reason to get me back home.

"No, Mama," I told her. "I'm not having it."

"What if you have one of those postabortion meltdowns?" she said.

"I won't," I said, trying to sound sure.

Really, my mother's offer was a formality. My father had recently quit drinking but my parents' marriage was unraveling all the same. The last thing they wanted, while they figured out how to walk away from twenty-four wedded years, was for their only daughter to drop out of college, pack up the whip-it canisters, and move home to raise a baby.

THE BURLINGTON BRANCH OF PLANNED PARENTHOOD scheduled abortions on Wednesdays only, when I had class all day, so I called a satellite clinic forty-five minutes away.

I had to put my name on the books regardless of my decision. The law varies, state to state, but there was (is) usually a limit to the number of weeks into a pregnancy a woman can terminate. Vermont had either the most lax laws in the country or zero available information: my online research yielded no results. In most jurisdictions, the process became more complicated or just illegal after thirteen weeks' gestation. I didn't know how far along I was—not more than five weeks, which was all the time that had passed since my first sex with Noah—or how long the wait for an appointment would be.

"Have you had a pregnancy test?" asked the receptionist.

"Yeah." Why? Did girls show up on a hunch?

"First available is three weeks out."

The end of April.

In the dining hall, I filled my tray with fried chicken to feed the baby protein and waited for Ruby to join me in a red leather booth.

"Wanna know something crazy?" I asked as she slid into the bench across from me.

"Crazier than a vegetarian eating meat?" She pointed at my tray.

"I'm pregnant." Her mouth fell open and her fork fell out of her hand. Eventually, her face snapped back into place.

"Friend. This is the worst," she exclaimed. "What are you going to do, put a crib in the dorm room? Feed with soft serve from the dining hall?"

"Have you ever heard of this happening?" I asked. "To someone who has always wanted children, is cheating on the love of her life, and swore she'd never, ever have an abortion?"

"Who'd swear such a thing?" she replied. "Sounds religious."

"What if I end it and go insane?" I chewed half-heartedly on a piece of chicken.

"It's probably the lesser of two evils."

She shook her head.

I shook my head.

We shook our heads.

I STARED AT THE WATER-STAINED CEILING from the vantage of Noah's bare mattress. I couldn't stand the insufferable mélange of symptoms: a permanent ice cream headache, even though I wasn't eating ice cream. A sudden aversion to my staples (marinara sauce, salsa, coffee, and red wine). I subsisted on bottles of Orangina and saltines. I crashed by 8 P.M. Noah turned over and grabbed a bottle of nasal spray from the carpet. He took off the cap and squirted it up his nose to enlarge his nasal passages, allowing OxyContin to take faster. He passed me the bottle.

"Really?" I snapped. I'd quit drinking and drugs to nourish the embryo that I wasn't sure I'd keep. The southern part of me wished he would get clean and return to college and work a legal job so we could have the baby.

Noah and I came from the same country, different worlds. In Massachusetts, a successful smear campaign would expose a politician for voting against abortion access; in Kentucky, a candidate would *win* an election for voting down access. In my world, you had the child. You married. My best friend's mother gave birth to her at age seventeen.

Noah muted the television.

"Do you want to have this baby?" he asked.

"We could call her Jade," I said. All eleven of my grandmother's siblings had names starting with "J." Mick Jagger had a daughter named Jade.

"Jade's pretty," he said. "But I'm not ready to be a father."

I TOOK DOWN THE PHOTO OF Will-B's newborn niece and stuck it in my desk drawer before Googling adoption agencies. I learned that millions of children around the world don't have permanent homes, don't have parents. There are 143 million orphans in developing countries alone. Five hundred and eight thousand children were in the U.S. foster care system that year; and that didn't include the babies adopted from birth.

WebMD, my trusted source of medical advice, informed me that I had unwittingly participated in nearly every activity that experts list as harmful to fragile beings inside the womb: binge drinking nightly, smoking weed and cigarettes, taking high doses of antidepressants, mainlining coffee, standing near microwaves, eating genetically modified foods, ingesting vitamin A supplements, getting my hair highlighted, swilling tap water, and jumping rope in the quad. In better news, I had neither handled reptiles nor dug around in a cat's litter box. So it could have been worse.

When adoption was off the table, I researched the emotional afterlife of abortion.

All I wanted was a bunch of women to sit with me in the same room and tell me they'd had an abortion—even though they wanted to be mothers and shared my moral qualms—and tell me how to get okay. After an hour of reading online, I felt like nobody would level with me. Everything I read registered as political propaganda.

According to antiabortion websites, abortion may cause alcoholism. May cause anorexia. May cause obesity, depression, anxiety, divorce, sex issues, hallucinations, nightmares about babies, fear of babies, obsessions with babies, quote-unquote maternal confusion—all symptoms of "postabortion syndrome," a term coined by a pro-life psychologist named Vincent Rue in 1981. In 1987, I read, the U.S. Surgeon General C. Everett Koop examined more than 250 studies to determine whether terminating a pregnancy ruins the minds of women. Given Koop's conservative Christian views, he was expected to substantiate the claim, but the medical studies failed to yield a reliable conclusion. While the news media portrayed the physician as saying there was no evidence of a correlation between abortion and mental health, that was misleading. In a 1989 letter to the White House, Koop wrote: "I have concluded in my review of this issue that, at this time, the available scientific evidence about the psychological sequelae of abortion simply cannot support either the preconceived beliefs of those pro-life or of those pro-choice."

So nobody knew shit. The studies had been too subpar to tell. Even Koop said he had counseled women who felt severely emotionally wounded and heard from others who'd touted the health benefits of terminating a pregnancy.

In 1989, the American Psychological Association, purportedly free of political influence (though, really, who was?), had convened its own team of experts to take a look at the available scientific studies. They'd determined that severe reactions were rare, most people handled an abortion much like other familiar life stresses, and yet others endured profound suffering. Newer scientific studies had been similarly inconclusive: a handful of them presented evidence that terminating posed no greater risk to a woman's mental health than childbirth, while another collection of studies suggested that abortion was uniquely dangerous to the mind.

According to some of the most reputable reproductive health organizations, abortion may cause relief. *And?* I wondered. These websites debunked abortion myths and explained that the "Anti's" were
inventing faux terminology to scare people off. While the information was medically accurate, it was also sanitized and incomplete.

I concluded that having an abortion would be a gamble: I'd either
lose my mind, or win a shiny future with a good husband, a master's
degree, and money to live well.

In search of other women who had actually terminated a pregnancy and had real answers, I brushed out my knotty platinum hair
and swept it up in a smooth, scholarly bun, to go to the library and
scan the shelves. I ducked down, knees to chest, whenever I heard
footsteps, paranoid that a classmate would see me and ask what I
was looking for: a memoir about abortion in the absence of an actual
conversation with a human being. No luck. On a sofa at the counseling center, I hugged my queasy stomach in front of a therapist with
wisdom creases around her eyes, praying she'd have her own story
to tell. She told me no story. Instead, she compared an abortion to
killing a bug.

One last place to check for answers: church. I had a wild idea that
a priest would miraculously intuit that I was pregnant and tell me
she'd had an abortion. I imagined this scenario even though I had
never seen a female priest before, even though I had never heard a
religious leader say the word abortion in the somewhat progressive
Episcopal church where my family had gone to get our holiday dose
of God.

Gripping the wheel of my salt-caked green Explorer, I drove cau-
tiously through the frozen valleys of Vermont toward a provincial
town of Massachusetts, where Noah's parents lived. I talked to the
thing in my belly, asking its input, begging for a sign, but all I saw
were road signs pointing to Noah's childhood home.

Under a white comforter in his king-size bed, I pressured him to tell his mother and father that I was pregnant. Part of me hoped they'd help raise the baby. Another part of me hoped they'd help fund the $415 procedure, since we didn't have the cash ourselves. But Noah felt he'd hurt them too much already and didn't want to add Knocking Up the New Girl to their list of his mistakes.

When the two of us headed out to church in the morning, his mother waved, holding open the glass door, saying, "I don't know what you've done with my son, but I like it." I smiled, too sick to feel guilty. I'd scavenged a black crochet dress from the trunk of my car. Noah sported his "court clothes," a navy blue sports coat and red tie. I didn't tell him I was putting myself in front of God hoping to hear a message that would make everything clear.

We slid into a pew that had to be as young as our relationship—no bored T-ball star's initials carved in the wood. Noah was surprisingly keyed into the sermon. In front of us, a newborn was slung over his father's houndstooth shoulder. Snap pea fingers, a pad of hair on his misshapen head. My heart shifted.

I waited to hear a disembodied voice booming inside my ears: KASSI. IT'S ME: GOD. GIVE THE BABY BACK TO ME AND GO BACK TO COLLEGE. THANKS FOR YOUR OBEDIENCE. DON'T BE A STRANGER.

But I heard nothing.

NOTHING EXCEPT A HARSH GRINDING HUM on the road back to Burlington, flanked by snowcapped mountains. Heat blew on my hands on the steering wheel. Noah slept with his head propped against the window. It wasn't him making the noise.

It was the engine. I parked in the dorm parking lot and jiggled the key in the ignition, but the clunker coughed its last.

We had fifteen dollars between us.

I was broke, jobless, nineteen, pregnant, 891 miles from home, with no transportation to the clinic 46 miles away. Even my foot was broken. I didn't qualify for a credit card. Bluegrass Family Health didn't cover the procedure. As far as being a "provider," Noah was the world's worst drug dealer. He had two clients: Minivan Dad and himself.

The message light on my flip phone was blinking red when I got up to my dorm room. "Kass, it's me." Will-B. "I feel like I'm having a relationship with your answering machine. Call me back, please. Lemme know you're okay."

I couldn't. I wasn't.

Surely Will-B would be shocked and astounded if he returned home after a yearlong tour in Korea to find me in a maternity dress with an orbed belly. I couldn't do that to him. I would make my pregnancy disappear and erase the evidence of Noah, try to preserve the possibility of continuing my relationship with Will-B and become worthy of him again.

I called my mother and told her that my car had broken down and my foot was broken, too. Then I went from dorm door to dorm door, asking any old body for permission to borrow a car for a ninety-two-mile trip. I found my coach: a blue Subaru. A couple of days later, a $400 check arrived from my mother with the words "car repair" scribbled in the memo line.

ON THE WAY TO PLANNED PARENTHOOD, Noah and I stopped by the bank. The teller scanned the check with his eyes and did his bank teller routine and then casually stuck it in the drawer and said, "It'll take about a week to process. K?"

"Actually, I need the cash now," I whisper-talked.

"It's against policy."

"I have a doctor's appointment in one hour and this check's paying for it."

"This is an out-of-state check," he whisper-mocked me. "We don't hand over four hundred dollars cash for out-of-state checks."

"Please," I whisper-begged. "I can't reschedule the appointment. I've been waiting for three weeks. I'm borrowing somebody's car and I can't go through this again. The appointment's in forty-five minutes."

"It's so against policy that I could get fired."

"Can't you call the bank in Kentucky and clear it with them? The check's good. It's from my mother."

He opened his drawer again and examined the check. The memo line read "car repair." He studied me for a minute. I studied him back. Hormonal tears fell straight down my face and I wasn't wiping them away. I wanted to tell him exactly what the money was for, but I think he knew. His cash machine dinged.

THE HOSPITAL GOWN WAS HIKED UP to my stomach, a blanket belted across my middle. I lay back, flipping through photographs from the March for Women's Lives in Washington, DC, two days earlier.

Ruby had ridden a stuffy bus there, trooped down the National Mall and DC streets, ridden back, and left the pictures on my desk that morning. More than a million people marched in Washington, and I had spent three weeks searching for only one woman to lead me through this—and had not found her.

The doctor pulled a monitor over that would have shown me a living thing in the splayed light, but I looked away.

"Don't tell me if it's twins," I said.

"Here comes the speculum," she replied.

The nurse offered me her hand, encouraged me to dig in with my fingernails.

I wanted to tell her that I had captained the cheerleading team in high school, edited the school newspaper, worked two coffee shop jobs when I was seventeen to save up for vintage fake furs. I was a good Christian, a virgin until last year. This was not supposed to be happening to me.

"I'm in the honors society," I said.

"You'll have a big life," the nurse replied.

The suction machine droned like a hair dryer.

"I'm blacking out," I shrieked.

"You've got to breathe, honey," said the nurse, giving my hand a squeeze.

"I'm hot. Please take off my socks."

"Take off her socks," Noah hollered. The nurse whipped them off.

Afterward, I curled up on the crinkly exam table paper. Somebody rolled away a table with a tiny red gob in a jar—my almost baby.

I shook violently, viciously. Sliding off the table in my hospital gown, I pulled my underwear halfway up my legs and fumbled with an inch-thick pad, trying to stick it on the crotch of my underwear. I tugged my bell-sleeve sweater over my head and then headed down the hall.

Somebody handed me a brown paper bag with three packets of birth control in it. Somebody opened the front door of the clinic for me.

I WOULD DREAM OF BABIES FOR the next six years: I would have babies and kill them, have babies and lose them, have babies and care for them the way I cared for my little brother. I would believe every reason for my abortion was absurd. I would nearly go insane. I would start my car and drive toward a psych ward in Texas and then turn back around. I wasn't insane. I was sad. I wished sadness took less work to heal, but healing would take everything I had.

- 3 -

CRAZY LOVE

ONE MONTH AFTERWARD—It hadn't felt to me like the traditional pregnancy I'd pictured, with the husband, baby showers, and retro maternity wear. But it wasn't *not* a pregnancy, either. I designed my own language to account for the nuance. I referred to this one as an "eggnancy," meaning a fertilized egg never meant to grow. I wanted to capture mine as a fly in amber. I became obsessed with womanhood and pregnant bellies. I referred to my abortion as "it," and "it" was constantly on my mind.

It was on my mind when I skipped my mandatory checkup at Planned Parenthood—"I can't come back here," I repeated to the nurse each time she told me it was required. I wish I had a firm reason why I couldn't go back, but I don't know—maybe I didn't have time to borrow a car and drive back again, maybe I felt too fragile to return to the scene of my abortion, or maybe I just didn't feel like it.

"It" was on my mind when I carried my two-hundred-pound orange floral couch down three flights of stairs with Ruby, parking it on the curb outside the dorm building; when I tore my vintage wardrobe off wire hangers, pitching clothes into two open suitcases; when I slipped the photos of Will-B, his niece, and the army of activists marching on Washington into a backpack.

Ruby switched off the overhead light. I shut the door that Noah had knocked on for the first time fewer than three months earlier, and we lumbered down the steps with our luggage.

"Don't look back," said Ruby, before sliding into the front seat of her father's sedan.

My flight to Kentucky would leave in seven days; Will-B's plane would land in the same airport a week later. I pictured him walking off the jet bridge in his military fatigues. I could feel my breath catching in my throat and was already up off my seat and running toward him. But this self who was running toward him wasn't the self I used to be.

Wearing the fifty-pound backpack, I trundled my two rolling suitcases along two miles of broken sidewalk until I reached Noah's front door. The dorm buildings were locked. The town of Burlington had cleared out as students returned to their home states to visit their parents before summer. I had arranged to stay with him.

Noah's roommate answered the door. A tall and cocky redhead, he wore ironed khaki pants and pastel plaid shirts and sold bags of heroin that he kept in his dresser. He stood in the doorway with his eyebrows raised and lips pursed, conveying his obvious displeasure at the sight of me.

"Noah's not here," he said flatly.

Noah had skipped town for a concert in another state, forgetting that I had nowhere else to stay. I asked his roommate if I could sleep in Noah's bed anyway.

"No way," he said, closing the door. It began to drizzle.

I marched furiously down the wet and weedy sidewalk, past the rundown clapboard houses on the north end. The rain fell harder. My two suitcases were drenched. I was drenched, mascara tears spilling down my face.

I couldn't tell my parents I was stranded in Burlington for seven days. They were already worried. Withdrawing me from UVM and moving me permanently back home felt like an imminent threat—and a bad idea, at least from what little I could gather. My mother had already said, "Don't tell Rusty about you-know-what. Your brother's got this idea that you're pure. I don't know if he'd talk to you ever again if he knew." "Ever again" was a long time, and I couldn't stop telling people about my abortion. Talking about it was keeping me sane.

So I went to the only person I knew would take me in: Dez—the boss from the vintage store who'd fired me, the only woman I really knew who'd decided against motherhood, a zaftig thirtysomething with spiked hair.

She opened the front door.

"I'm not pregnant anymore," I told her. The rain beat on my head. Tiny rivers dripped from my split ends down my soaked blue ski jacket. My suitcases were parked behind me, the pack heavy on my back. She opened her arms and I fell into them, hit with the reality of it all. She stroked my wet hair and let me stay with her until my plane took off for Kentucky.

But the home I returned to only vaguely resembled the one I had left.

I recognized the three blooming white dogwood trees on the front lawn on Strawberry Lane, but the house was quiet and missing furniture. I'd go to sit down on a chair and find it wasn't there—it would be in my father's new house on the other side of town, where he moved when my parents separated.

Exhausted, I walked through the halls by myself, flanked by empty places on the walls where pictures used to hang, toward my bedroom to curl up in my familiar bed. I opened my bedroom door and discovered a patch of dented brown carpet where my childhood bed had been. It was gone. The fishnet canopy fell straight down and pooled up on the floor. I swallowed the stone in my throat.

The reunion with Will-B didn't happen after all, either. Not after I ran into his buddies gathered at the counter of a local bar downtown.

"You and Will-B? Really? He never told me that you were together," said his cousin Hock, an old friend and classmate, a mixed expression of pleasure and disbelief under the blue brim of his baseball cap.

"Yeah." I felt my face redden and sink. "Since, like, last June. A year."

I silently ticked down a mental list of evidence that we had, in fact, been together: his family photographs. Letters. Emails. I wanted to pull my phone out of my corduroy handbag and scroll to a voice message from him.

"Hey-y-y-y-y," his friends yelled in unison while I slammed a shot they'd bought me in celebration, faking a delighted laugh while my insides curdled in humiliation, thinking, *I'd rather be stranded in the rain with two suitcases and a fifty-pound backpack than standing in this bar, claiming to be Will-B's girlfriend of a year to his friends who've got no clue.*

So I took an early return flight to Burlington. I looked sternly out the plane's oval window at the fluff of clouds. Will-B must have been crossing the ocean in his army fatigues while my plane hovered thousands of feet above the horse farms.

The only way to move forward was to go back.

I WAS IN THE BACKSEAT OF a car southbound on I-89 from Burlington to Tennessee heading for the Bonnaroo Music and Arts Festival. Noah was pale and tinted green, his chin on his chest. I was holding a balled-up tissue to his nose to keep the blood from dripping on his plain white T-shirt. Rain drummed on the car roof, the windshield. The driver, in front of me in a baseball cap, bobbed his head to Phish's "Free." Every half-hour, Noah crushed up OxyContin pills and snorted earthworm-size rows of powder off the vinyl album cover of the Grateful Dead's *Skeletons from the Closet.* The cover art features Venus, the caramel-haired Roman goddess of fertility, a man behind her and a skeleton in front of her.

I thought Noah was on the verge of an overdose and so I kept poking his nose with my pointer-finger-wrapped-in-tissue to stop him from dozing off. I could never tell whether he was sleeping or dead. Before we'd hit the road, a heavyset girl standing at six feet and dressed like a skinhead in plaid pleats and Doc Martens had appeared in his den. She and I made small talk and then I returned to Noah's bedroom. Five minutes later, I heard a *THUD*. I tried to ignore the *THUD*, but there was no subsequent movement, nobody picking up whatever had fallen down. By the time I found the girl, she was lying unconscious on her back and not breathing. Her lips were purple. A syringe was on the floor next to her. I screamed and Noah darted in past me and squatted behind her, picking her up by the armpits. He propped her up on her knees and hung her front-ways over the back of a chair. He slapped her right cheek so hard it echoed, shouting her name. At some point I dialed 911, my hands shaking violently, but Noah commanded me to hang up. I followed his instructions, pacing back and forth, praying she would survive. After three minutes of slapping, the girl came back to life.

But I couldn't forget her purple lips. I monitored Noah's mouth in case he showed signs of losing consciousness. I couldn't bring him back if he ODed. I didn't know how.

I wondered whether he thought about the abortion every waking millisecond like I did, whether feelings, any feeling, poured through him like sludge, but I didn't want to trigger him to use more by bringing it up. I pressed two fingers against the radial pulse of his clammy wrist.

The driver dropped us off at the edge of a farm that backed up to Bonnaroo. Noah and I climbed out of the car with our backpacks and paid the farmer twenty bucks. Tents were pitched as far as the eye could see, clustered into villages. We pitched ours, green and shabby, its threads twirling in the breeze. I crawled inside to make a bed out of blankets and backpacks while Noah jumped a fence into the festival to search for the porta potties. I checked my watch to mark the time he left. Four P.M.; I'd give him twenty minutes before I started to worry.

Thirty minutes later, he wasn't back. Calling him, I listened to the phone ring into an abyss.

Forty minutes passed.

Voicemail.

Fifty.

Voicemail.

Fifty-five.

Fifty-seven.

Voicemail.

Voicemail.

When Noah had been gone an hour and fifteen minutes, I went from tent to tent, describing his appearance. Glassy hazel eyes, long-ish black hair, Phish T-shirt, a missing-persons sketch that was as specific as "combat fatigues" would be at an army base.

We hadn't bought tickets for the festival. The green paper band around my wrist was counterfeit, the creation of a woman wearing a fairy costume in a Walmart parking lot, where we'd stopped earlier. She colored strips of paper with a neon green marker, labeling them with the word "Bonaroo," misspelled with only one "n."

I set one sandaled foot on the farmer's fence and hopped over. The music festival looked like the end of the world. A unified mass of fig-ures wearing dusty clothes, carrying backpacks and water pouches and babies in slings, all moving in the same direction. I folded into the crowd, straightening out my embroidered halter-top every few steps. The bass beat vibrated in my cells. Bright red nitrous balloons were handed down to me from the back of a semi-trailer truck. I held the end of the balloon to my mouth and sucked it until my brain crackled like a sparkler and then snuffed out. I called Noah again. Voicemail.

I staggered through the matted brown grass and opened porta-potty doors, expecting to find him slumped over a plastic commode with a syringe sticking out of his arm. *Bang-slam. Bang-slam.* No Noah. He had to be dead.

I felt too fragile to handle another catastrophe fewer than two months after the catastrophe of getting pregnant and having an abortion. I imagined Noah's wake, his funeral, sitting at his mother's kitchen counter and not telling her that I could have had his child.

Back at the campsite, I sat down in the tent, bum in and legs out, with two beers sloshing all over my hands. Then, in the distance, I saw a figure in the field walking toward me. His sneakers slapped the ground like a pair of flippers.

"Noah," I screamed. I leaped to my feet. "Where the hell have you been?"

He reached into the pockets of his shorts and pulled out two handfuls of long green authentic wristbands, maybe fifty of them in each fist.

Over the past three hours, he had persuaded a Bonnaroo employee to take a break and let Noah wear his staff T-shirt. In uniform, Noah greeted cars in one of the many lanes at the entrance where festival-goers arrived and exchanged printouts of their tickets for an official Bonnaroo wristband. While he handed out green wristbands, he also stole as many of them as his pockets would hold.

During his "shift," a black SUV with a Kentucky license plate stopped in his lane. The windows rolled down. Five guys filled the seats. "My girlfriend's from Kentucky!" Noah told them.

Of the thousands of cars that delivered ninety thousand people to Bonnaroo, one of them, one that stopped in Noah's lane, of all the lanes to choose from, was packed with my and Will-B's buddies.

"Who's Will-B?" Noah asked me. He sat on his haunches next to me, smoking an unfiltered Camel.

"I don't know," I lied. "I don't know who he is."

This answer seemed to satisfy Noah.

He sold the wristbands for $100 a pop in the Walmart parking lot, bagging $2,000 in cash before midnight. I was proud of him for being resourceful enough to stage a heist and earn money by selling items that didn't belong to him.

It was 1 A.M.

"Here," said Noah, handing me a stack of twenties. "I owe you half of that four hundred." He had his head down. "I'm really sorry," he said, facing me, but not looking at me.

"Don't be," I said, not sure how to respond because I wasn't sure what he was apologizing for.

"I should have known what I was doing," he said.

"No, Noah. Please don't blame yourself," I said, reaching out to take him by the arm. He scrunched up his face in a grimace and ducked into the tent. I wanted to ask him whether that was why he was using so much, but didn't want him to feel criticized for using.

I bought ecstasy with the abortion money from Noah. Blissed out, we climbed over the fence and headed toward a fuzzy glow of orange lights strung up around white tents at the craft market. Noah bought me a silk peasant top and sticks of incense and never-ending love beads. A rhinestone headpiece. A loose black velvet skirt. I felt like we were rich people. I fantasized that we could grow up and have a normal relationship and a new Jade as divine compensation.

But then I lost him in the crowd, and when I eventually found him he was totally obliterated, pitched forward and staggering around in a circle in the mud. He'd lost a shoe. He slung one arm over my shoulder, propping himself up on me as we stumbled back to the campsite.

IN BURLINGTON FOR THE REST OF the summer, I moved into a dilapidated Victorian house with five other girls, one freestanding bathtub, and a kitchen nook stacked three feet high with used-up boxes of wine and empty cans of Pabst Blue Ribbon. The couches were draped with college students and drifters who wore glitter on their brow bones and dreadlocks stacked on their heads. The walls were half-painted turquoise, because somebody got sidetracked and just gave up.

I sat on the rundown front porch, alone with a glass of vodka and *The Red Tent*, a novel my roommates passed around like a secret recipe that summer. It imagines the women in the Bible coming together during their menstrual cycles for fellowship, encouragement, and stories. I wished we had a monthly gathering like that for women who had had abortions.

I weighed barely a hundred pounds. My dirty hair was hitched up in a messy bun, my cutoffs and halter-top were grimy after months of chasing Noah—trying to prevent him from falling asleep with a lit cigarette in his mouth, engulfing the mattress in flames; cooking him chicken dinners to supplement his diet of Ensure and gummy worms (he never ate the meal); stopping up his nose bleeds; channeling any leftover maternal instinct into him. His parents had just taken him away to a ninety-day drug treatment program in southern Vermont. Ashamed that I hadn't been able to get him clean myself, I saved his rehab phone number in my cell as "Noah—Summer Camp."

I flipped through *The Red Tent*, finding peace in my paperback and drink. I marked up the sun-dappled pages with a pen, picturing my foremothers gathering together, telling stories. I carefully underlined the passage, "If you want to understand any woman you must first ask about her mother and then listen carefully," doubting that it applied to me. I thought I had little in common with my mother. With

a Kentucky twang, she had told me, "It's not too late to be a debutante in white." I turned her down—at my debutante ball, we'd all
wear red. Still hell-bent on motherhood, I wanted to leave a record for
my future daughter so she wouldn't mistake terminating as a sign
of weakness. "Until you are the woman on the bricks, you have no
idea how death stands in the corner, ready to play his part. Until you
are the woman on the bricks, you do not know the power that rises
from other women—even strangers speaking an unknown tongue,
invoking the names of unfamiliar goddesses." "On the bricks" meant
childbirth. I crossed out *on the bricks* and scribbled *having an abortion*.

My flip phone buzzed. Will-B's name lit up the screen.

"Will-B," I said. He said he'd been stationed in Fort Drum, New
York, 205 miles away from me. He was currently driving those 205
miles to Burlington. Shit.

"I need to tell you something," I said, not knowing where to start.
"It's not good," I warned him.

"It's okay, Kass," he said, perhaps knowing what I would say—at
least some of it—and not wanting me to say it.

I started with the first truth. "I'm seeing somebody else," I said.
"I'm sorry. I'm so sorry I didn't tell you sooner."

I explained that Noah had left town for a long vacation, that it was
pretty much over with him.

"I'm alright," Will-B said. "I mean that's alright. I still want to see
you."

I wanted to see him, too, pretend that the past six months hadn't
happened and pick up where we had left off—with my plan to graduate college and walk down the aisle to him and exchange vows on his
father's farm back home.

"Meet me at Ri-Ra on Church Street," I told him. The Irish pub
where I was currently working was the only place that hadn't fired
me yet.

I shaved my legs, rubbed foundation on my face, and brushed loads of mascara on my eyelashes. I spritzed my wrist with Chanel Chance, the perfume I had sprayed in the packages I sent to Korea. I felt for the first time since April that I could recalibrate. I was twenty years old now and could have been five months pregnant, but instead I was zipping up a pair of high-heeled boots and going to work. And meeting with Will-B as though Noah didn't exist.

I sold bottles of Guinness out of a stainless steel tub on a table positioned inside near the entrance of the bar. A couple of hours later Will-B appeared in front of me, looking a little lost. I jumped off the stool and into his arms. He dipped me back and planted one on me. He put his hands on his hips, wearing a needlepoint belt lined with jockey silks.

"I stand out here, don't I?" he yelled over the loud talk and house band. Will-B's voice was more comforting than my missing bed at home in Kentucky. We ducked under my table and took shots of Patron tequila. Will-B loved Patron. Yelling the word "Patron," pronouncing the word "Patron" in various accents, consuming Patron in large quantities. When my shift was over, we walked home together with our arms around each other. I couldn't wait to get drunker.

On the front porch, Will-B, my artillery ammunition specialist army faux-hawked lover, passed the bottle around to my five antigun, antiwar, anti-Bush roommates until we were staggering around in the streets yelling *Hooah!* and *U.S.A.! U.S.A.!* Eventually, the girls grew tired and filed inside, the screen door slamming shut behind them.

Will-B and I sat on the front steps, staring at the street. The blue light of dawn rolled over the painted Victorians. Birds began to chirp. He scooted closer to me. I kissed red stripes down his cheek. He scooped me up from the bench and carried me to the bedroom.

I had kissed his mouth at every age for six years—fourteen, fifteen, sixteen, seventeen, eighteen, but skipped nineteen and jumped to twenty. The only year we hadn't kissed was the year we were committed, the year I got pregnant by somebody else.

He pulled up my shirt and kissed my stomach on his knees. Stunned with guilt, I grabbed his belt buckle and unbuckled it. He returned to my mouth. He reached up my skirt and pulled my underwear down to my knees.

"I don't want to have sex," I blurted out.

"Okay," he said, stopping, hovering over me, studying me intently. "Ever?"

"Not *ever*." I intended to explore one-night stands and random encounters with other men—but I wanted to be sacred to somebody. Even if I messed up everywhere else, there could be this other reality, the one where I was a paragon of virtue. In *Fear of Flying*, Isadora Wing had an extramarital affair and still ended up with her husband. I could have it both ways, too—experience the lusty exploits of a philandering girlfriend and a side pregnancy with a kid who knocked me up fewer than two weeks after I learned his name. Then, preserving my ideal of domestic perfection, I'd still marry the stable, caring, patient, loyal, true, psychoanalyst next door. Will-B wasn't a shrink, but he had the right disposition and a tendency to psychoanalyze, pointing to our similar fathers as the cause of our bond that was both intimate and distant.

I wanted to press the pause button and return to this moment in five years, by which point I hoped my hair would have stopped falling out in the shower. And I would have acquired a thing called dignity.

OVER THE NEXT TWO MONTHS, Will-B breezed in each weekend, befriending my roommates and classmates. The Vermont crew was obsessed with the hippie-soldier-horseman I brought to parties, with his Kentucky turns of phrase and bottles of Patron. I watched for a hurt look in his eye or a turn of phrase that might suggest his heart was broken, but he seemed completely unfazed.

I wasn't going to let him know that I'd had a conniption and left town when I found out he had hidden our long-distance relationship from his buddies. I couldn't let him think I was desperate by asking him why he hadn't taken us seriously enough to tell them.

It was an election year. Will-B and the girls lazed in the den, watching a presidential debate. They sipped wine or tea from an assortment of mismatched mugs. I sank into a couch cushion after a cool jog under the gold autumn trees. I tucked one knee to my chest to untie my shoelace. Will-B had slid halfway down his seat on the couch and was balancing a water bottle on his chest. A politician talked about his campaign to defend the life of the unborn.

"That's what you do when you have an abortion," I said to the television. "You protect the unborn."

From my peripheral vision, I could tell Will-B was now looking at me. I kept my head down, my ponytail falling over my shoulder, untying my other shoelace, slowly, methodically, thinking now was as good a time as any to tell him. Because there is no good time to tell a guy who already knows that you cheated on him that you had also became pregnant with someone else and had an abortion. There is no good time to tell someone who is more than a boyfriend, an old friend, a good enough person to drive 410 miles back and forth each weekend to hang out with you even though you're partly drunk and partly in love with him and partly committed to a mysterious person somewhere else and partly have no idea how to get out of the f*ck that has become your life. There is no better time to tell the truth than now.

"Why do you think that's what an abortion is?" he asked.

I peeled off my socks and told him why. Then he wanted to know when. I told him when.

It wasn't fair, but I wanted Will-B to be a hundred things for me in that moment. I wanted him to comfort me. I wanted him to carry me upstairs while I hugged his neck and cried on his shoulder because of what I had done behind his back. I wanted him to let me apologize.

Will-B shook his head as if to adjust to the new information, stuck in this den with six women, with nowhere he could go to process it without making it obvious that he'd been affected by it, if he had at all.

Some of my roommates stared into their cups. One closed her eyes and pretended to be in a distant state of meditation.

"I thought you wanted to be a mother," he said, his voice softening.

"I do," I shot back.

"I thought if you got pregnant, you'd keep the baby."

I wondered whether he would have wanted to.

"I thought so, too," I said.

I hastily gathered up my sneakers and socks and leaped up the staircase, hoping he would follow me, but he didn't. I nudged my bedroom door open with my shoulder and hurled both sneakers at the wall as hard as I could. I paced across the floor with heavy steps and picked up my sneakers by their laces and threw them at the wall again. I heard the screen door slam shut downstairs and thought I would never see him again, but he had only stepped out on the porch to smoke a cigarette below my window.

We wouldn't speak of it for ten more years.

A MONTH LATER, WE WERE ON OUR SIDES, facing each other in my bed with the lights turned out. I told him Noah had been in rehab, not on vacation, and now, at this very minute, he was on a Greyhound en route to Burlington.

"So I need you to go to the couch," I said, tipsy enough to be direct but not drunk enough to feel no remorse. "I'm scared he'll relapse if he finds us." What I meant was, *I'm scared he'll die and it'll be my fault.*

"Kass," Will-B said, as if to say, *Don't do this.* He grabbed me gently by the shoulders and pulled me closer to him, as if I should read his mind and know exactly what he was thinking without his saying it out loud. Maybe I could, but I wanted him to say it.

"I'm sorry," I stammered, shaking out of his grip.

He rolled over on his back and sighed a sigh that became a groan and filled the room.

"He won't know. As soon as he gets here, I'll leave," Will-B said. I didn't want him to persuade me to stay with him for a night. I wanted him to fight for me to be with him.

He swung his legs over the bed, swiped his khakis from the floor, and pulled his pants on with one quick jump. He quickly buckled his belt.

"I could hide in your closet," Will-B suggested, starting to mess with me. "It's big enough to sleep in. Don't you think?"

I stood up next to the bed in my underwear and crossed my arms over my chest. He scanned the shadowy floorboards, then grabbed his balled-up shirt from the corner.

"Or," he continued, "I could crawl under the bed. They taught us these moves in the army. Just like the trenches. I could crouch down with your sewing machine and old photographs. I'll just open the window and jump out."

"Why did you have to come here at all?" I yelled. "You knew I had a boyfriend." I wanted him to unleash, grab my candlesticks and throw them against the wall, tell me he loved me to my face and not from the other side of the planet.

"I wanted to see if there was anything left," he said, and walked out of my room with a soldier's posture, buttoning his shirt, the tails fluttering in his wake.

When the sun came up through the blinds, Noah was sleeping next to me, strands of his black hair stuck to his cheek, dried blood under one nostril. Barefoot, I hopped out of bed.

An envelope had been slipped under my door. My name was chicken-scratched on the front. I tore it open and pulled out a two-page note:

Kassi,

I expected you to be madly in love with me, but you are not. When I came home from a year in Korea, I thought you would be one of the first people I laid eyes on, and we would go into the amazing love affair I had been dreaming about every night for the last year. But that is all it ended up to be, a dream. It is heart wrecking to see you with another guy, but no matter how much I have thought about it, we will not have a crazy love affair, and even though they would be damn good looking, we won't have kids. Your happiness lies in someone else's heart. I have come to terms with that. And as awkward as it makes me feel, sleeping on the couch while Noah is with you, I have accepted that, too. Although I think I'm better than the guys you hang with, I realize that is my little stupid opinion, and I'm probably not. I hope I can fool another girl as attractive as you are to fall for whatever I am. But one thing I know to be true about myself is that I am a great friend. I would never turn my back on you or be reluctant to give up anything for you. I love you.

See you in Kentucky.
wBVm

"I love you" looked like it was an afterthought, the letters squished together like a group of old friends crowding together for a photograph. The ink was a paler shade of black, as though he had gently applied pressure to the pen to scratch out those words before he stuffed the letter into the envelope—just in case I wanted to chase after him and apologize and beg him to take me back. I did want to, but I knew that even if I drove the 205 miles to his army base and clasped my hands together and vowed to change, I would turn around and drive back as the same person who had cheated on him and stopped answering his phone calls while she figured out what to do about an unwanted pregnancy. I didn't want to be her anymore. In the hall, backed against my bedroom door, I pressed my cell phone to my ear.

"He's high," I said to Noah's mother.

"Kick him out," she said matter-of-factly, so used to her son's addiction. "He may never get better. Move on, Kass. If it's our permission you need, then you've got it."

"I'm afraid he'll die," I told her. I could have been eight months pregnant.

"He might," she said. "But we can't stop living."

I hung up and stood over Noah, watching him sleep for a minute. I nudged him on the shoulder. "You gotta go," I whispered. He had to go because I had to change.

Meeting me in the doorway, he ran his hand through my hair. I stared at him, expressionless, my stomach dropping. He would cycle through rehab and jail and a halfway house and his parents' house. Noah was never coming back. Our baby was never coming back. With so much not coming back, I had no reason to stay.

- 4 -

THE BATHROOM IS MY
PRAYER TEMPLE

EIGHT MONTHS AFTERWARD—I scooted into my window seat on
the plane with a Nalgene bottle full of wine in one hand and a travel
brochure in the other. The brochure came from an office at the university where I had washed up one afternoon and examined a stack
of glossy pamphlets fanned out on a small table. I selected one with
a pink cathedral on the cover. It read: STUDY ABROAD IN FLOR-
ENCE ITALY.

I opened the accordion brochure on the plane.

"Going somewhere?" asked a man who was settling into the seat
next to me. He was smooth. He was handsome and black, eyebrows
straight across, oval-shaped glasses. I didn't know that he was a leg-
endary poet whose name I would hear and whose face I would see
plastered on university bulletin boards forever thereafter—that,
twelve years later, a poster of his face would be tacked to the glass
window of the bookshop below my apartment.

"Italy," I replied, taking a swig from my Nalgene bottle. I was half-
drunk with half-moons of mascara under my eyes. "I had an abortion and now I'm going to Italy."

Taboo had no power over me because taboo meant nothing. I

talked about my abortion with anyone, everywhere. I talked to persuade myself that it really had happened. I talked because I didn't
want another woman to feel as alone as I had felt. I denied I needed to
heal because that four-letter word didn't contain the same definition
for me as others might infer. Having an abortion did not break me.
It revealed the ways I was already broken. A lush with panic attacks
and skimpy self-esteem, a well-meaning liar with a fear of being stupid. It also revealed the traps set up for women that made us tuck
in our wings and die when we're still alive. The media got abortion
all wrong. Women who had terminated their pregnancies were not
frail and wounded little sparrows. Having an abortion was not for
the faint of heart. For thousands of years, women had possessed the
strength to protect themselves and their children from a world that
couldn't hold them both, only to be portrayed as depressive mur-
derers. Having an abortion had affirmed my love of life. I longed to
expand—to be loud and wild and uncensored. I just couldn't pull it
off without a drink. Part of me knew I would have to learn how to be
brave without whiskey and wine. Maybe it was the same part of me
that wanted a circle of women who could teach me how to fly at full
wingspan and shake up the established order of things.

I found no support group in the classifieds, on the counseling
center bulletin board, or anywhere else. I couldn't articulate what I
needed because it didn't exist. It felt unsafe and destabilizing to admit I needed something that simply wasn't there—people who'd had
an abortion coming together regularly to plunge the depths of the
wound and bring out power from the void. Sometimes we cheated
on the people we loved, got knocked up, had an abortion, and then,
the very next morning, put on lipstick and a blue dress and walked
to class.

"Italy after an abortion, eh?" The man smiled. He seemed to be
getting a kick out of me. "What's the plan when you get there?"

To buy my own liquor, for one thing. I met the legal drinking age in Europe but had to depend on my twenty-one-year-old friends in the United States. They had put an embargo on supplying my alcohol and planned an intervention that I had sidestepped by boarding this airplane. I scanned my brochure for a noble answer—and saw classes in women's literature.

"I'm a writer," I said, by which I meant I was an English major. "And a feminist," I added. "My abortion was my feminist awakening."

"Is that right?" he asked.

I nodded. "I'm going to read Italian feminists and write a book about my abortion," I said, surprised to hear myself make such a statement. Authoring the book I couldn't find in the library was the first idea that had given me a sense of purpose in a long time.

"You ought to write that book," said the man. Then he took off his glasses and held them in his lap, closing his eyes while he reclined in his seat.

When the plane landed in my layover city, the man asked, "What now? On to Florence?"

"No." I was such a sham. "I'm just heading home for Christmas."

I didn't even have a passport.

HOLIDAY LIGHTS WERE STRUNG UP IN the trees in my hometown, and then the branches were bare again, and it was just winter, just January. I didn't have a plane ticket for Europe, but I was waiting on a rush-ordered passport. Each day I intended to secure a student loan and sign up for the program and search for Italian living quarters, but day would turn into night and night would turn into morning and morning would turn into another day gone by that I had done nothing to further my plan. The evenings blurred together in a montage of waitressing at a local diner, getting fired from the diner, and falling down drunk in the grass with a random townie.

At 6 P.M. on an evening much like the others, on the way to pick up carryout dinner, police pulled me over on Euclid Avenue. I parked in the bike lane with the blue strobe lights flashing behind my car. I didn't feel too drunk to drive but doubted the cop would agree with me. I knew my spike heels and taupe 1940s coat with the fur collar were attempts to create a diversion from my bloated face and permanently bloodshot eyes.

I failed the Breathalyzer test. The cop pushed me into the backseat of the cruiser to the tune of blaring police sirens. He manacled my wrists behind my back, cinched so tight they cut my skin. I maneuvered my hands into the pocket of my coat and pinched a penny from the shredded lining. I managed to stick the penny in my mouth so I could suck on it, remembering an old wives' tale that sucking on a penny could foil a Breathalyzer test—as if a penny in my mouth could change the result of a test I had already taken.

In jail, a man in an orange jumpsuit with a teardrop tattoo under his left eye delivered me a lunch bag containing a baloney sandwich like the ones my father used to make (sans mustard smiley face). A friend posted bail around 6 A.M. Doing nothing during nine hours in jail mirrored the nothing I had done the nine months before I was arrested. I didn't have an abortion just to fritter the hours, accomplishing nothing. I wasn't just wasting one life anymore—I was wasting two.

My father, who had been sober for more than a year, pulled up in front of the Strawberry Lane house wearing a baseball cap embroidered with the words "Heart of the Bluegrass," the brim forced into a geeky upside-down "V." The curls around his face had paled into gray. His round face sagged more with each of my visits home. He had begun to look like many men. I often thought I saw him in airports or on city streets.

"You look sick, Moto," he said as I climbed in, avoiding eye contact. There was no mirror on the passenger's side of his truck, but I knew what I looked like: his pale and puffy daughter, with a swollen, aching liver, in a baggy gray sweat suit after a long night in jail. In Vermont, there was a warrant out for my arrest for an unpaid noise violation I received during a rowdy house party. In Kentucky, I had a lawyer, a court hearing, and a driver's license that had just been revoked for DUI. I was twenty years old.

"I am not trying to be hard on you, Kassi. We are all very worried."

"I need to go to Italy," I solemnly replied. My passport had arrived in the mail while I was in the clink.

"You'll be lucky to survive the week at the rate you're going," he said.

We were stopped at a traffic light. I stared gravely at the road ahead.

"Would you please take me to the Italian consulate in Detroit?" I said, maintaining composure with all my might. The drive was five and one-half hours each way. "I need a student visa. I checked online and there's a three-month waitlist, but I think we can persuade them to stamp my passport if we show up in person. My program starts in a week."

"You've got to be kidding me."

"I won't drink," I said, a storm front of hysteria.

Dad released a nervous laugh in disbelief but agreed to take me to Detroit on the condition that I read a letter written by Carl Jung, the founder of analytical psychology.

Jung had addressed it to Bill Wilson, the author of the "Big Book," the urtext of all Twelve Step programs, the "instruction manual" for Alcoholics Anonymous. I agreed to read the letter, though I was surprised. The only text I had ever seen my father read had been the *Daily Racing Form.*

We printed out the MapQuest route to Detroit and the missive from Jung. We swung by a gas station and stocked up on water and chocolate, known to stave off cravings for alcohol. Then my father set out to drive me 344 miles north to the General Consulate of Italy.

The sun flickered through the frozen bare trees outside the car window, a strobe light on the page I held in my hands. In a letter dated January 30, 1961, Jung acknowledged that alcoholism was misunderstood: the "craving for alcohol was the equivalent on a low level of the spiritual thirst of our being for wholeness, expressed in medieval language: the union with God. How could one formulate such an insight in a language that is not misunderstood in our days?"

Equating my desire for Gordon's vodka to a desire for God didn't sound primitive to me; it sounded useless. I wasn't mad at God, even though "please don't let me be pregnant" had been my one and only college prayer, or for being busy the day I sat in a church pew with an embryo in my belly, waiting for a sign, or for not stopping Noah from sticking heroin needles in veins. God just had a bad track record for showing up. I couldn't imagine a divine entity making me feel as content as alcohol did, or why I would crave union with a God that, as far as I could tell, wasn't available to perform miracles much less to say hi.

My father persuaded the clerk at the consulate to stamp my passport with a visa.

Jung goes on: "The only right and legitimate way to such an experience is, that it happens to you in reality and it can only happen to you when you walk on a path, which leads you to higher understanding."

Wishing Jung would just bullet-point the higher understanding, I secured a $20,000 loan and booked my flight to Italy.

"You see," Jung continued, "Alcohol in Latin is 'spiritus' and you use the same word for the highest religious experience as well as for the most depraving poison. The helpful formula therefore is: *spiritus contra spiritum*."

Spirit against the ravages of the spirits.

One week later, the wheels of the plane were up. I was on my way to Florence.

WHEN I CALLED MY MOTHER three weeks into my five-month study abroad program, I had burned through my loan, maxed out my five thousand dollar credit card limit, and was living off €100 I had borrowed from my new roommate, an American Orthodox Christian virgin who had the misfortune of being assigned a twin bed opposite mine. Tina displayed a bottle of holy water on her nightstand, sprinkling her head at bedtime. I had holy water, too: a bottle of Chianti. I left a voice message for my mother, imploring her to pay down my credit card.

At the Internet café down the street, I found an email from her waiting at the top of my inbox with the subject line, It Didn't Take Long. The message riffed on how *it didn't take long* for me to ruin my fresh start. She had spoken to my father over the phone, and they had agreed to front me seventy euros a week, which would barely pay for a seven-day supply of pasta and canned marinara sauce.

Twelve hours later, I sat in a windowless bathroom with an empty tequila bottle between my legs, rolling around in my palm a new key chain—a translucent bust with a pink plastic embryo floating inside of it. This was not the first night I had drunken a bottle of tequila alone in the bathroom of my flat, but it was the first time I really wanted to stop—at least for a couple of days. It was not my tequila. It was Tina's tequila, which I had repeatedly stolen and then replaced. I had traveled halfway around the globe to outrun myself, and here I was. Still me, and not me at all.

I pressed the cell phone to my ear and listened to it ring across the ocean.

"Daddy?" I said, trying to sound casual.

"Is that you, Kass?" I must have sounded bad. I was, after all, his only daughter.

"It's really hard to quit drinking," I said. "I don't think I can do it."

Within minutes, my father had me on the phone with a sober American who lived nearby in Florence and attended English-language Twelve Step meetings. Her directions had me wending around several crowded piazzas under the bluest sky I had ever seen, through an ornate black gate, down a walkway to the side door of a church, and then down a spiral staircase to the basement.

When I began my 1.7-mile walk, I had no intention of quitting drinking permanently—just long enough for my parents to trust me and to replenish my funds and for my cough to go away and my bruises to heal. Wandering past the bearded accordion players and marble statues, I picked up my pace—and suddenly, inexplicably, I never wanted to drink again.

I bumbled into the basement room wearing a belly-baring shirt and the same 1940s box coat I had worn in jail in Kentucky. These ex-drunks knew exactly what to do: they sat me down in a purple child-size seat and fed me sugar cookies and gathered round the long table to tell their stories. I looked at them: a plump Englishwoman in a faded floral housedress, two American twentysomethings, a Latino-American artist with a lip ring, a white ultra-Catholic painter dressed all in black with tattoos swirling around his arms. They refilled my coffee cup and dumped another helping of baked goods on the plate of sweets I'd already scarfed down.

They talked in a language I could understand: "Alcohol worked," said a woman. "Then it stopped being fun. And it was just sad." *Amen,* I thought. A man in a white scarf and business suit said, "I was breaking my standards faster than I could lower them." I cracked a smile, though I had to wonder whether my standards had been particularly well conceived in the first place.

I was mystified that I was turning myself in to a bunch of sober dorks in a church basement, but everyone else was doing the same thing. I wished somebody would talk about ending a pregnancy, but it would be years before I heard a woman weaving the story of her abortion into her sobriety tale from the podium, and that woman would be me.

"David," said a deep British accent that belonged to the man who'd settled into the chair across from me after the meeting. Completely out of sorts, I reached out with my left hand to give him a shake.

"I'm David," he said again, not as puzzled by my left-handed greeting as I would have been.

"Hi," I said.

Dressed in a collared polo shirt, he looked like he wore sunblock year-round and appeared to be in his mid-forties. He was excruciatingly kind. I could tell he was religious, and somehow that was all right with me. A navy blue softcover book came sliding across the table toward me.

I recognized the text. While my college friends opened packages filled with socks and cash, I had received from my father the Big Book, six months before I got pregnant.

The point of the instructions in the blue book, David explained, was to connect me with the divine power deep down within myself. It almost brought tears to my eyes, insofar as I allowed myself to be affected by such promises, to think that there was anything divine about me.

David suggested it would help to align my mind with loving thought: to pray.

He prayed each morning—on his knees.

"I'm a feminist," I said. "That sounds submissive."

"It is," David answered.

I crossed my arms in defiance, but for some reason, I was relieved.

"Don't quit before the miracle happens," David said as I ascended the spiral staircase after the meeting.

Walking back through the piazzas, I peered through bug-eye black sunglasses, my hair a sprawling blonde mess, my jeans too tight, my shirt too short. I fastened the chunky buttons on my coat. I considered the weight of the book in my hand. *My God,* I thought. *My life is over.*

SEVENTY EUROS IS PLENTY OF MONEY when your life is over. It's hard to complain about detox when your life is over. When your life is over, everything that happens is a miracle and nothing else exists. In fact, I should start every morning with this prayer: *My life is over.*

I stuck with the group in the church basement. Swayed by my progress in recovery, my mother Western Unioned me a little extra money. Three weeks after my last drink, I set off with Tina and my backpack, riding trains through Austria and the Alps and the south of France and then on to Paris.

At Bercy train station an enormous man wearing an enormous black suit told us of a two-star hotel that cost only as much as a hostel. His name was Edward. He worked as a scout for Hotel Belford, telling tourists like Tina and me about a discounted rate.

Seated on the crisp hotel bed, I riffled through my purse. My passport was missing. I searched the pockets of my coat, opened all the zippers of my backpack, checked the tabletops. I called the front desk, who called the train station. Nobody had turned in a stray passport.

Without a passport, I couldn't go anywhere—not back to Florence, not even back home.

I had inconvenienced Tina since the day we had met two months earlier. I woke her up at all hours, spilled red wine on her UGGs, stole her tequila, borrowed €100 that I still owed her. She deigned to take a chance on me, a newly sober travel companion, and I up and lost my damn passport. Tina could have been strolling through a gilded Hall of Mirrors or visiting Jim Morrison's grave, but instead we were rushing around Paris trying to fix my latest mistake.

At the U.S. Embassy, a security guard with bushy eyebrows was locking the gates. It was Friday and we had to leave Sunday. The embassy was closed until Monday.

"Can you make an exception?" I begged. "I don't have the money to stay here until Monday and I lost my passport. Please."

"No," the security guard replied.

I apologized profusely to Tina as we shuffled through the streets, the cars circling us in the wet dark night, lights flickering from tall green lampposts. I had ruined Paris.

I left Tina under the Eiffel Tower and ducked into a restaurant bathroom, remembering David's suggestion to pray on my knees. I locked the stall door and knelt down on the blue and broken tiles. What I really wanted to do was curl up and cry on this bathroom floor, but instead I clasped my hands together. To the tune of "All I Need Is a Miracle," I prayed for a passport miracle. For a clue. I wasn't giving away my power so much as humbly empowering myself with a power that worked. An answer came. Maybe it was from God, or maybe from a better part of me.

And it wasn't what I expected. God didn't tell me the geographical coordinates of my passport. The message was this: *Girlfriend, you are stuck in Paris, not in jail. Get up off your knees and have some fun with Tina.*

I found her by a lamppost. It began to slush torrentially. Holding our purses over our heads, we belted out "All I Need Is a Miracle" at the top of our lungs, following the wide and glinting streets in the direction of our hotel. We fell asleep to the murmur of French television.

The next morning, the phone *brrrrrred* with a wake-up call I had not asked for.

"Is this Kassi Underwood?"

"Yes," I said, my eyes still closed.

"Kassi, this is Edward. Your passport was turned in at the train station. Come quick. Be here in twenty minutes or they'll send it to the U.S. Embassy and you'll have to wait until the end of the weekend. Come on, girl!"

Tina and I bolted out of the hotel toward the train station. At the end of the platform, there was Edward the giant, jumping up and down in his black suit and waving his hands over his head. We sprinted toward him until we slammed into his towering frame in a group hug. We cheered and jumped up and down with him.

After that, bathrooms became my prayer temples. I would kneel down in bathrooms everywhere, some of them at thirty thousand feet cruising altitude, but I spent the next three months praying in bathrooms all over Europe. Turns out, the opiate of the people is some good shit.

For now, in Paris, I thanked the God of Lost Passports. I thanked all the gods.

MY MOTHER TRAVELED TO EUROPE FOR the first time, ever, to spend some time with me. She was ready to take on Italy.

I was exhausted after three months of what sober people called "the work." The path to a higher understanding that Jung described wasn't what I had expected. As far as I could tell, spiritual clarity was a by-product of emotional and mental clarity (or vice versa), which was the by-product of finite tasks, like listing my fears, grudges, and sex conduct on paper in a specific format. "The work" hadn't brought me to a higher understanding of my abortion, but there would be time for that later. At the moment, I wanted my mother, but "Daughter Collapsing in Arms" was not listed on her itinerary.

Mom and I wedged through the crowded doorway of the Duomo, the cathedral in the center of Florence, the earth within the earth. A Mass was under way, and the other tourists whispered to one another. A fuzzy column of light fell on the marble floor.

"Wow, Kass," she repeated, as we walked around the yawning cathedral. Her southern accent bounced up the walls. She kept saying
she was happy to "have me back." Last time we had been together,
she'd cried all the way to the airport, and not because she was going
to miss me.

We filed behind a line of people into a stuffy narrow stairwell
and walked up and up the spiral tunnel. Neon graffiti splattered the
walls with names ending in vowels. I followed my mother's echoing
voice. She chattered all the way toward the roof of the Duomo, losing
her breath and then beginning again.

We walked out of the dark stairwell and onto a platform that circled all the way around the base of the dome. Over the railing was a
hundred-foot drop to the backs of travelers kneeling for Mass on the
marble floor. Nursing her lifelong fear of heights, my mother turned
away from the guardrail and latched onto the wall, spider-like.

"Ma?"

"Yeah?"

"You okay?"

Her whole body shook. She held her neck stiff and her hands to
the wall, as if ready for a shakedown. A line of sightseers formed
behind us.

"Tell them to go around," she said in a strained whisper.

We made ourselves flush while I waved people by. I put my arm
around her shoulder. She relaxed into my embrace, with her cheek
pressed against mine.

"I don't think I can do it," she whispered to me.

She sounded put out with herself, but I cajoled her into letting me
act as a buffer between her and the edge. We crept to the foot of a
staircase that spiraled to the lookout point.

"You go. You go on," she said, turning her head halfway to me, her
cheek flat against the wall. Her forehead was slick with sweat. Her

apple green shirt clung to the small of her back. Little by slowly, she inched into an alcove and stood next to a security guard who blocked her view of the long drop down.

"I'm not going up without you," I said.

"I said, go." There was a hint of anger in her voice.

My mother had taken me to the edge of the opening, pushed me as far as she could. I gripped the cold railing and climbed skyward through the dark by myself.

ONE OF THOSE POSTABORTION MELTDOWNS IN WHICH I QUESTION MY PLACE IN THE AFTERLIFE

THREE YEARS AFTERWARD—I was sitting at a desk in an office in Texas, dressed in high heels and a pencil skirt, editing books about fraud. Chewing on bubble gum, I scanned the screen inattentively, sliding my eyes across an email from Noah. I expected an update on his attempt to kick heroin. He wrote that he'd met a girl at a music festival. They'd managed to stay together during his stints in jail.

She was six months pregnant with their daughter, whom they'd named Jade.

None of my other exes had children. None of my girlfriends had kids. Nobody I knew my age had a child except, now, the last person in the world I had ever expected—the father of the baby I had aborted, who had told me he wasn't ready to be father.

I locked myself in the office bathroom and dropped to my knees. The tiles were whirling. Prayer has a way of humbling me to the truth, so I didn't pray. I was afraid that God would say that I had murdered my own child, even though I didn't think abortion was murder. I thought, *I should have had the baby.* Then I thought, *It wasn't a baby. It was cells. Products of conception.* Jade. I lay down on my back and tugged at a fast-spinning roll of toilet paper, handfuls of it in my hands, and stared at the vaulted ceiling. I wanted to die, but I wasn't allowed to die because I might go to hell.

"I GUESS I SHOULD TELL YOU that I had an abortion." The word now felt cumbersome in my mouth. Larry, my new therapist, said nothing, just looked at me from his swivel chair. I continued: "Isn't this information, like, part of the intake?"

Larry bobbed his head. "Anything can be part of the intake, Kassi."

By the time I became his patient, I had been sober two years, turned twenty-two, graduated from college, and pointed my compass south-bound down I-89 toward the retro postcard town of Austin, Texas, with its rivers and lakes and pinup girl bangs, its honkytonk song-sters, all long in the vowel and frayed in the sleeve. I was hired as a writer and editor for an antifraud education company. I funneled money into two retirement funds. I watered my plants. I waited pa-tiently for Will-B to finish dating someone else. But a haze had set-tled over me, and my mind would not shut up.

Larry was an addiction specialist. The addiction in question was my abortion. I was addicted to pregnant bellies. To my translucent bust key chain, with its floating pink embryo. To the one-inch giraffes and pirates and plastic diapered babies displayed above my key rack at home. I wanted to end the constant thoughts of my termination without telling anyone other than Larry that such troubling, impos-sible thoughts occurred to me. I was supposed to be head-butting glass ceilings, not ruminating on a baby that would have obliterated my plans. I was also supposed to serve others as part of my sobriety, to avoid guzzling cooking sherry and Listerine. The classic feminist argument held that abortion wasn't selfish, but that idea now seemed suspect, like a ridiculous generalization meant to give me a false sense of peace. Because I suddenly realized that I could have had the baby. And suddenly, for the first time in my life, I was afraid of God. God: not a man in the sky, but shorthand for the indefinable power that kept me sober. Alive.

The wooden blinds in Larry's office shut out the Texas sun. Thermometers reached ninety degrees. Florescent overhead lighting carved a black shadow in Larry's gray head of hair. He had a Caesar haircut, a neat 'do I imagined he brushed with the slim comb on his desk. The room was cramped with stacks of papers and books. I shifted my weight on the leather couch.

In therapy sessions, my abortion was like an empty black box, an object to be noted: sharp corners, a shiny, forbidding exterior, nothing inside.

"Well, Kassi, how do you feel about the abortion now?" Larry was a chronic name-user.

"Fine, I guess. I never thought I would get pregnant unintentionally, but when I did, the choice was fairly obvious. He's still addicted to heroin. Anyway, I'm here because my brain is attacking me."

AT WORK THE NEXT AFTERNOON, I sipped a mug of coffee and proofed *Fraud Magazine*.

The exam table, the nurse's hand.

The digital clock pulsed to 2 P.M. In loopy black handwriting, I scrawled "Congratulations!" on a sticky note, stuck it to a box of diapers, and crossed the blurry parking lot, filing into the Fraud Museum behind my colleagues for a baby shower.

The exam table, the nurse's hand, the hum of the vacuum.

My co-worker had the resigned expression of an expectant woman near delivery. I smiled and said I couldn't wait to meet her little one. "Go on, feel it," she drawled. She grabbed my wrist and flattened my palm on her belly. "That's his head," she told me.

My baby had a head.

I sliced a wedge of sheet cake and sat down on a stool in the corner of the room under a framed photograph of Houdini, who devoted his career in magic to making people disappear.

"Speech, speech," a few people chanted to the pregnant woman.

I lie supine, rest my cheek on the sticky leather.

"Get this little shit out of me so I can drink again!" She smirked, stuffing a forkful of cake in her mouth.

The doctor takes a pair of rubber gloves from the box on the windowsill. Noah touches my shoulder.

I had read that depression could be caused by allergies, but my allergist didn't think so. In appointments with Larry, I surmised that maybe I was depressed because of the antifraud company, which had rejected my petition for a subsidized onsite daycare that would benefit the new mothers pumping breast milk in the bathroom, retroactively give me options, proactively prepare for another accident. Or maybe it was because of my dalliance with a doctoral student who said his Roman Catholic parents would never accept me because of my abortion. Planning my future, a life that would have been seemingly impossible if I had been a young, broke, addicted, single mother, had always been a balm on my brain. But now I shuddered when I jotted my new goals on a sticky note. My plan was suspiciously grandiose.

"Do you think I have narcissistic personality disorder?" I asked Larry, hugging myself on his couch. He shook his head with a knowing smile. No, he said, I was merely a person in my twenties.

"Kassi, you need to trust yourself," he said, over and over. I didn't know how to trust myself because I wasn't sure I was trustworthy.

I blurted out to Larry that I could feel the baby in my throat.

"The body remembers," he replied.

———————

NOAH'S JADE WAS BORN IN EARLY FALL. I couldn't stop thinking about the baby that wasn't, a loss suddenly made more painful by the baby that was. I spent my workdays browsing photos of Noah's little girl on Facebook, believing I was somehow glimpsing the face of the child we could have had. In her baptism photos, Jade puffed out her cheeks like a blowfish. I went home to cry in bed on my lunch break, longing for a paranormal miracle. I had somehow convinced myself that Noah's new baby was a replica of ours. I felt a sense of ownership, of responsibility for the child's happiness. But I couldn't tell Larry—he'd think I was crazy.

At my next therapy appointment, I entered his office and dropped my purse and sat down on his leather couch in a full-blown panic attack about the baby I feared I had killed.

"I can't breathe," I said. "I need to cancel and go home."

I didn't move.

I press my heels into the stirrups, can hear the heartbeat on the monitor.

"Kassi, try to stay," said Larry. "You can just lie there on the sofa and focus on your breath."

"How am I supposed to focus on my breath when I can't breathe?"

"Kassi, you need a meditation practice."

"Please, just tell me what's wrong with me." I choked back tears, was embarrassed for him to see me cry, for him to know that my thoughts were so unbearable that I wanted to be institutionalized. Yet, I couldn't tell him that I was thinking about dying because then he might institutionalize me. Nothing made sense.

"Do you think I'll go to hell?" I asked. I wasn't sure I believed in hell, but I knew I did not want to go there.

The metal speculum is burning cold, the cone-shaped rods sting, my cervix is dilated.

"No," Larry replied, but I didn't believe him. I couldn't banish the thought: I had taken a life.

JUST BY LOOKING AT ME, it would have been hard to tell that I worried about eternal damnation. I was promoted at the fraud business. I had a white male assistant and a new car on the company dime. I had a thick black streak in my blonde hair. I wore earrings so big you could serve bread on them. I strutted around the office in four-inch heels. On lunch breaks, I dined with friends at restaurants with yogic names like House of Light, where we talked about our financial advisors. Evenings, I jogged with a glamorous jet-setting colleague who was as unstoppable in her career as I hoped to be. I hosted girls' nights and piled into cars with a bunch of braless chicks with hairy armpits and headed to Ani DiFranco concerts. I could hardly admit to myself that my depression had anything to do with deferring motherhood, let alone to my progressive friends who perceived suffering after an abortion as a myth constructed by the conservative religious right and believed only by women who didn't have minds of their own.

Some of them had had abortions, too, but we didn't talk about them. We talked about conservative male politicians trying to snap up our rights. Looking back, I spent too much time shit-talking those politicians and not enough time acknowledging where I fell short in my respect for other women, including those who had an abortion and then protested against them. I *am* that woman, I thought. I just happened to be holding a different sign.

In a study titled "Abortion as Stigma: Cognitive and Emotional Implications of Concealment," researchers Brenda Major and Richard H. Gramzow found that keeping an abortion a secret was correlated with attempts to suppress thoughts about it. Ironically, suppressing the thoughts triggered even more powerful thoughts like the ones shooting through my skull. My secret wasn't that I had an abortion;

everybody knew about that. My secret was that it had been a big deal, that I wasn't sure mine was the right decision, that I was afraid to live the life my abortion had granted me, afraid to fly at full wingspan, and I felt I was going mad.

At the gym, I thought I heard someone whisper my name. When I realized nobody had, I spent the next hour on the Elliptical with my face in a grimace, listening for other auditory hallucinations, convinced I was in the throes of a psychotic break. I consulted WebMD and then called Larry to recommend diagnoses that I both hoped and feared would land me in the psych ward.

I thought about meditating, but figured meditation would happen to me naturally: without my concerted effort, I would unexpectedly find myself sitting in the lotus position. Plus, my cynical side enjoyed making fun of the hifalutin new agers who meditated. Praying to God had become a thing I used to do, like playing laser tag stoned in high school. Prayer suddenly seemed like a gateway drug to religious zealotry that would alienate my friends and make me unapproachable to the people I needed: people who'd had an abortion.

One night, riddled with panic over the death-birth of Jade, I crossed my bedroom toward the restroom, where I had planned to splash my face with cold water and take my pulse. The next thing I remember is waking up on the shag rug next to my dresser with a throbbing chin. To prove to myself that I was alive, I sprung up off the floor and rushed over to my mirror, touching my jaw as I examined the brown marking. Then I lost consciousness again and came to on the floor with a gash in my forehead from the mirror's framed edge. I showed up at work the next morning with a purplish-yellow bruise on my jaw and a fresh scab that protruded from my forehead like a walnut-sized third eye.

"How's the other guy?" asked my colleague.

I told him I was the other guy.

That night, when I walked through my kitchen, I froze: knives. I was afraid of knives. I was afraid I would slit my wrists without my own permission.

The doctor rolls away the instrument table, the blood-filled jar with a pea-sized brain inside of it.

With nothing else to try, I gave meditation a shot. I unzipped my pencil skirt, opened the shower stall, and melted to my knees. Water snapped against the tiles. I tried to find my breath, but I still couldn't breathe. I stayed there for what felt like an hour but was probably three minutes. Maybe meditation wouldn't work. Maybe nothing would.

When I slept at night, a baby boy floated in front of me with a pole for a neck, floating up into the sky where I feared he wouldn't survive in the atmosphere, but I couldn't catch him in time. A drowned girl stared at me from underwater, her yellow hair radiating like limp sunrays.

Another visitation came from a teenage boy, tall as a beanstalk with extra-long arms. "Mom," he said, "Mom, remember me?" When he morphed into a Japanese boy, I assured him I wasn't his mother. Then, suddenly, I remembered that I was his mother after all and apologized for forgetting him. "You can't be my mother," he said. "My true mother lives in Manhattan."

I thought that Manhattan could cure my depression, so I surfed the website of the graduate program in creative writing at Columbia University. Columbia's landing page, an aerial view of the domed arctic blue rooftops and grassy quad, warmed me with the faintest glow of hope.

My undergraduate thesis advisor, a bespectacled memoirist with a mountain man beard, had filled my arms with paperbacks from his bookshelf—Joan Didion, Lauren Slater, and Anne Lamott—and encouraged me to apply to Columbia. My thesis had been a personal narrative about my abortion, a story I had chosen to end when I typed the last line, *I'm still alive,* though now that Jade had been born, I wondered who that sentence was really about.

WHILE I WAITED TO HEAR BACK from my application to Columbia, I tried every available method of healing I could think of. I decided to correct my karma and make amends to my baby by becoming vegan. Cutting all animal products from my diet, I filled my grocery cart with soy peanut butter ice cream, tofu chicken fingers, and Oreos (naturally vegan). I would save the lives of sentient creatures while testing my friendship with anyone who had the misfortune of dining with me.

Even though my brain burned wild with sorrow over the Jade that was and the Jade that wasn't, even though I sat through meditations with a brick in my heart and static in my head, I hoped changing my habits would change the way I felt. In the mornings, I dropped to my knees to pray on the bathroom tiles. I prayed impersonal prayers to a businesslike God. I was afraid. I was afraid that if left a vulnerable opening, God might say the only sufficient reparation was celibacy. Then I sat on the toilet seat to meditate for a grand total of five minutes, occasionally losing focus and nibbling on almonds or checking People.com.

I made friends with a man named Greg, and not just because he was a dead-ringer for Tom Cruise in *Top Gun.* He introduced me to other people as a writer, even though I hadn't published a thing. Greg was thirty-six, I was twenty-three. He dressed like a '90s slacker in plaid pants thinning at one knee. I liked his sense of humor. He emailed me to say, "Slept ten hours last night. It was amazing. I think I'm ovulating." We sat under the Texas sky on the wrought-iron chairs at Spiderhouse, a coffee shop decorated like a yard sale. Greg riffed on the outdoor gnome statues, speculating on what the gnomes did when the shop closed down at night, while I doubled over with my legs crossed, literally wetting my pants with laughter. Larry the Therapist had told me that when I met a healthy man, I'd initially think he was gay or uninterested. Check.

Greg directed a home shopping network called the Jewelry Channel overnight and dashed off funny articles for me to peruse during my nine-to-five workday. One was an article from the satirical newspaper *The Onion* titled "Rock-Bottom Loser Entertaining Offers from Several Religions."

I cracked up reading the article at work, but I also thought, *That's not a bad idea.*

When I told Greg I was trying to meditate, he whisked me off to a Buddhist meditation center called Shambhala. In a starch-white room, people sat in rows, straight-backed and cross-legged, on cushions called gomden—the Tibetan word for meditation cushion. It was so official, so comfortable—I had to have one of my own.

After some online sleuthing, I tracked down a gomden at a small shop in Vermont called Samadhi Cushions. The package with my new cushion landed on my Austin front porch the next week. I tore the navy blue cushion out of the box and took it to the bathroom, placing it on the tiles in front of the toilet. I sat down on the cushion. It was firm, not lumpy. It felt familiar to me, like sitting on a horse. I could do this: I could become A Meditator.

Not long afterward, my cell phone buzzed with a call from a private number. I ran to the office kitchen to answer it. A professor from Columbia invited me to join them in the fall.

I spent the next week in ecstasy. I wanted to move to New York since I was a little girl—and never had this dream involved bringing a three-year-old baby with me. Really, the only detail in the dream was walking down the street. In middle school, my friend Charlie and I used to deck out in all black with spike heels from her dress-up closet and sit out on her farm, puffing on cigarettes. Affecting Fran Drescher accents, we'd say, "So I was walking down the street," because that's what people did in New York. Walking down the street would have been good enough for me, but becoming a "writer" seemed like lotto luck.

Greg texted his congratulations. "Of course you're in. I'm so happy for you. But selfishly, I'm sad."

Although I wanted to remain his friend, I also wanted to kiss him. One chilly winter night, under the isolated beam of streetlamp in a restaurant parking lot, we hugged our usual ambiguous goodbye and then I laid one on him. He kissed me back, but not as passionately as I had hoped. The next night, we were lying side-by-side in my bed, completely undressed.

"New York, huh?" he said.

I unloaded: "I'm in the midst of a meltdown. I got pregnant when I was nineteen and didn't have a baby. I thought I was fine. And I was fine, but the guy who didn't want the baby with me just had a baby with someone else and I can't stop thinking about it. Sometimes I feel like I'm on the brink of madness. Nothing seems to fix it. Maybe New York will."

"Are you on birth control?" he asked, jerking his head toward me, cocking one eyebrow with a frightened look in his eyes.

"An IUD," I said. He slowly lowered his head back down to the pillow. I wanted to say, *I'm not crazy!* but he had already made his judgment.

"I've always thought it was bullshit that women have to act like nothing happened after an abortion," he said. "It's their prerogative not to need anything afterward, but to have to choose between being harassed for talking about it and keeping it a secret . . . reminds me of soldiers coming home."

Other than Larry the Therapist, Greg was the only person I had told about the meltdown, my hope for a geographical cure. A thirty-six-year-old Texan whom I'd known for six months had supplied me with the closest analogy to having an abortion that I had ever heard—I felt I had "come home" to a country that misunderstands both its war and its "soldiers."

Greg tucked one hand behind his head, his elbow in the air.

"I think that happened to me, once."

"You knocked somebody up?"

"Yeah, fifteen years ago, college in San Francisco," he said, perhaps trying to sound casual. "A girl I was dating barged into my dorm, said she was pregnant and demanded a couple hundred dollars. I walked straight to an ATM and shelled it. Rumor was, she lied for drug money."

Brilliant fraud. "Did you ever ask her about the rumor?"

"Nah," he said, perhaps being the kind of person who would rather not know.

"Greg, I need to tell you something."

"What?"

"I'm pregnant," I joked. "I need four hundred bucks."

BEFORE THE BACK WINDOWS OF MY car bulged with garbage bags full of my clothes, before I passed through rough-hewn Texas towns lined with stores selling saltwater taffy and Stetson hats and drove toward the sparkling monster skyline of New York, I asked Noah to meet me for coffee.

I had flown to Boston for a fraud conference.

I was twenty-three, Noah was twenty-four, his Jade would turn one in the fall. Facebook pictures showed her to be a chubby thing with auburn ringlets. Her father had been bouncing around the local jails and borrowed a car from a kid at his halfway house to meet me.

Standing on Newbury Street in a navy business suit, I dabbed on a dusty pink shade of lip gloss. With a miserable smirk, I remembered that it was called Love Child. My hair was hitched up in a bun. My camisole clung to my back, dampened by the heat of summer.

Noah ambled up to the corner with his splay-footed strut. His puffy white Adidas smacked the pavement. Gone was his shaggy hair and mischievous smile. He had a prison shave under his sideways hat. His teeth were browned from drugs. Faded black tattoos sleeved his arms. We hugged. I muffled an unexpected yelp of sorrow into his smoky shirt.

We sat down for cappuccinos in a café where we could afford nothing else. He said paramedics had recently resuscitated him after he had overdosed in a Starbucks bathroom. Rehab followed. Now he scrimped by on construction work. His parents had adopted his little girl. I felt an urge to run to his parents' home and cradle his baby in my arms.

"I think a lot about what happened," he said.

"Me, too," I replied.

He stared ruefully into his steaming mug.

"But," I continued, "if I'd had that baby, you wouldn't have Jade."

Something was lost, but he got to keep it.

"Oh yeah," he said, flashing a relieved smile. To me, his smile meant something more. The abortion was mine alone, just like Jade was his.

"ROCK-BOTTOM LOSER ENTERTAINING OFFERS FROM SEVERAL RELIGIONS"

FIVE YEARS AFTERWARD — My purse vibrated. I wrenched my cell phone out of the faux leather sack and read the name on the screen: Will-B. (!) I was twenty-four, the age my mother had been when she wed my father, sitting by myself on the floor in a palatial library with two million volumes, surrounded by hardbacks on Buddhism. I stared at the phone in my hand, allowing it to buzz awhile so I didn't appear too eager. The lights in the stacks automatically switched off.

"Hey," I said into the glowing receiver.

"It's me," Will-B said.

"Hey me."

I had hardly seen him since he'd started courting a brunette banker named Sarah.

"I'm in Midtown," Will-B said. "Wanna grab a bite?"

It is poor form for a woman to accept a dinner invitation from an ex who is spoken for, especially when the aforementioned woman considers the aforementioned ex her beloved, her one and only, the one she has been waiting to come back to her.

I snatched my bomber jacket from the floor and threw it on midstride, en route to meet him at a restaurant on Broadway, wondering why he was in town, what this call was about.

IN THE FIVE YEARS SINCE HE'D slipped the letter under my bedroom door in Vermont, Will-B and I had checked in periodically to take the temperature of the relationship. The night my flight had landed in Lexington after my Italian sojourn, we'd dined downtown at an Italian restaurant. I had been eager to fix my mistakes with him and to reignite our romance now that I was sober for a whopping one hundred days. With no formal preparation, no serious thought, I had expressed my regret about "everything that happened when I was a drunk" with a tone that would have been appropriate for missing drinks on a buddy's birthday—when the reality was, I had cheated on him while he was serving in the military and had become pregnant.

"Stop," he snapped, shooting me a dead look. "That's not how you do it. You don't blame it on alcohol."

"Sorry," I said.

"No," he blurted out, as if he were answering a question I hadn't asked.

That Thanksgiving, I was putting a plate of turkey and corn pudding on his placemat and pouring him a glass of red wine, surrounded by my extended family, and my aunt asked him when he was going to pop the question—something I still hoped would happen when we lived in the same state. In the meantime, I decided to give him space and started dating a waiter, which I awkwardly explained to everyone present at the table. Will-B quickly finished his plate of food. When he left, I was sober enough to wonder what the hell was wrong with me.

I couldn't figure out why I couldn't get over him. By traditional standards, he didn't qualify for such persistent affection: he wasn't my first boyfriend, or first kiss, or first sex, or the first guy to tell me he loved me. It broke my heart that he didn't hate me. And if he was willing to get back together after knowing I'd been pregnant, then maybe I could have had the baby. So I kept him close, but pushed him away, always hoping we would get back together but afraid to live in a reality in which having had the baby seemed remotely feasible.

When Sarah entered Will-B's picture, he faded out of mine. My Facebook newsfeed resembled a gossip magazine: look at the bronze celebrity couple lounging in swimsuits under palm fronds, the happy duo attending a Kentucky Derby party (she donned an oversized sculpted red hat). Will-B emailed me on occasion to stay in touch, but I situated my replies firmly in the friend zone, trying not to feel what I felt for him. On Sarah's watch, he had stayed out of sight for three years.

BY THE TIME I HAD MOVED from Austin to New York, I shuttled underground in subways and hailed cabs with a flick of the wrist and speed-walked in boots. I thought about love, I thought about my abortion, unaware that my two preoccupations would soon become one.

I had a schedule packed with spiritual practices to maintain the appearance of stability, "appearance" being the key word. Prayer helped me to align with my better nature. I regularly ducked into the bathroom stall between classes to kneel down and beg for sanity. Meditation helped me to train my mind, by which I mean it leveled the playing field with normal humans. Inventorying my thoughts on paper helped me to make like Joan Didion and "find out what I'm thinking, what I'm looking at, what I see and what it means." I was building a mental shelter against intrusive thoughts. I walked carefully over the floorboards of my existence, as though stepping on the wrong plank, thinking one wrong thought, making one wrong move would destroy me and everyone close to me. Somewhere in the foundation was a bomb. I just didn't know where.

It was my contention that in order to avoid slipping into my past self, drinking until I developed early stage cirrhosis of the liver, cheating and lying, getting pregnant in a zipless romance, going broke in a foreign country, and losing my mind over my abortion, nothing short of perfection was required. If I breathed wrong, I would blow my life apart.

I took a course in Columbia's Religion Department to sneak some enlightenment into my literary curriculum. In the library, as I researched my final paper for Tibetan Buddhist Auto/Biography, I could almost feel the four-year-old ghost daughter standing at the end of the aisle with watery brown hair and porcelain skin, watching me blaze through books.

I CLICKED ACROSS CAMPUS IN black knee-high boots and saw Will-B waiting down a ways with his arms crossed. He had transformed from soldier boy to farm boy in a collared shirt and baseball cap with soft brown sideburns. The dimple on his chin had sunken in deeper. I gave him a big, obvious hug. He grabbed me by the shoulders, pulled me close, and planted a wet peck on my cheek.

"You look like your mom," he said.

"Thanks," I said, not sure what to make of it.

My mother had been trying to persuade me that Will-B and I were destined for each other. (I didn't tell her I agreed.) "I didn't much like him in high school," she'd drawl, "but the army made a man out of him. He came back from Korea, and I ran into him at the pool. I'd been so worried about you. He came over and gave me the biggest hug, and I told him, 'Will-B, you go up to Vermont and bring my baby home.' And he said, 'Yes ma'am, I will.' And I just knew I was looking at my son-in-law. He drove up to Vermont every weekend for you. He would've done anything. And you snubbed him for that druggie. Twice!"

"You've made it, Mama Kass," Will-B said now, putting his arm around my shoulder at the entrance to Columbia, before the black gates and stone statues of philosophers.

I wanted to think I had.

Will-B had earned a degree in equine business and was apprenticed to a famous horse trainer. By Kentucky Derby standards, that meant he was second in line to the king. He traveled the country to race thoroughbreds. In other words, he worked with expensive, unstable, and unpredictable creatures all day. That, I thought, is a man who could handle me.

On the way to dinner, I guided him down the twinkling tree-lined street to my brick prewar apartment building, situated on a corner across from the fire department, and pointed up at my eighth-floor bedroom window. Will-B tilted his head back to look and then lowered his eyes to meet mine and settled them there for the length of time before two people kiss for the first time, when both of them size up the situation, but then the eye contact went on even longer. It became a staring contest while cabs gunned by and the fire bell rang. I had my hand inside my purse, my index finger looped around the ring of keys to my apartment. Will-B moved toward the door and leaped up the front stoop. I wanted to take the key out of my purse and open the door and ride the elevator up to my bedroom with him and stay there with him until further notice.

What I did instead was work out an equation that went something like this:

The Buddhist in my head said: *Desire is suffering. It's the Second Noble Truth. Just stop wanting him and you will be happy!*

+

The single-minded career-driven feminist in my head said: *Don't go upstairs! You'll fall in love with him and sell out to the patriarchy and then you'll follow him back home. Don't give up! You had an abortion to achieve more!*

+

The sober person in my head said: *Warning. Danger. A man in relationship is an unavailable man. Do not ruin another woman's life just because you don't like yours. You'll drink. You'll die.*

=

Keep walking down the street.

The truth about why I didn't go upstairs was closer to a sappy sentence somebody had underlined in my paperback copy of Milan Kundera's novel, *The Book of Laughter and Forgetting*: "She loved him so much it would kill her, she loved him to the point of being afraid to make love with him because if she were to make love with him, she would never be able to live without him and she would die of grief and desire." I'd been afraid that someone would catch me reading it and think that I had underlined the passage so I snapped it shut real quick.

Will-B and I walked on toward the restaurant, and for years to come, I would wonder what might have happened if I had taken the key out of my purse and let myself fall in all the ways a girl can fall.

Seated outdoors at a two-top, I became oblivious to the commotion of pedestrians and traffic as Will-B quizzed me about everything from my old roommates in Vermont to my family dog. He talked like his jaw had come loose from the hinges, which looked like cocaine jaw, but wasn't. He had natural wisdom. I felt like I was made of plastic. I grew painfully aware of my all-black getup, red lipstick, bleached platinum hair with a black streak, my sparkly writer's dream, the product of bulldozing into whatever stood between me and what I wanted, but I still hadn't let myself have him. If the story had played out another way, would we have been together six years now, a traveling bohemian horse couple, training thoroughbreds and writing on the road? I pulsed with desire for that life and then smacked it down, I didn't know what it would take to live at full wingspan, the way my abortion had called me to live. But maybe it wasn't about a

business card and a white male assistant and an Ivy League education. Maybe living at full wingspan meant something else entirely. At
the moment, I felt so terrified to learn that my story could have been
different that I couldn't let myself feel what I felt for him.

Even my spiritual practice had become a mechanism for avoidance
as much as a path toward peace. I felt an explosion lurking below my
tranquil meditations, like I was wrapping a bomb in velvet with each
breath.

As dinner went on, I started to imagine a centerpiece on the table,
like an annoyingly tall flower arrangement that blocks your view of
the person seated across from you, but it was a baby, and I couldn't
move it out of the way, because it didn't exist anywhere except in my
mind. I realized I could never let myself be with him until I dealt with
my abortion.

I presumed that Will-B understood all the shit that had just worked
itself out in my head over on my side of the table. The plan was, I had
to go figure myself out. In the meantime, he would enjoy himself, date
the gorgeous banker, and wait for me to get my act together.

I emerged from my reverie hearing Will-B tell me that he had
bought a house in an area of Lexington populated by newlyweds.
Sarah wanted him to wrap his traveling horse enterprise and return
to Lexington. They would settle down there, marry, and breed.

I set my fork down on the table so I didn't stab myself in the neck.

"That's cool," I lied. Had we or had we not made an implicit pact to
play the field until we were ready to get back together? Was he telling
me this so I could stop him?

"So are you going to settle down?" I asked, my leg twitching under
the table.

"Yeah. I am." He shifted his eyes to the tablecloth. "Because I love
her."

I heard myself say, "I'm so happy for you. Sarah's amazing."

I drifted into a brownout, spoons clanking against bowls, echoes without words. I think I laughed on cue. Will-B flagged the waiter with a subtle nod, scratched out his signature on the check and then ducked into a taxi. The silhouette of the back of his head in the rear window made him look, for a brief moment, like anyone. But he wasn't anyone.

The next morning, I woke up with a raging fever. A ray of sun was crossing out my face as I blinked in bed, clutching the covers around my neck. Will-B had Sarah. Noah had Jade. I had a swollen throat and was swallowing razors. I had a gnawing sorrow in my solar plexus and hyper-awareness of my uterus when I thought of the abortion. The ex who had impregnated me was the father of a new baby girl, and the guy I thought I would marry was ending up with someone else.

I SLOGGED ACROSS CAMPUS IN SWEATPANTS and green Chuck Taylors, shivering, offended by the sapphire sky, the bleating taxicabs, holding my rolled-up final Buddhism paper. I had somehow contracted mono, the "kissing disease," which was a funny joke on behalf of the universe. After knowing Will-B a decade, he and I had hardly done more than make out and cause each other persistent disease. I told myself all sorts of things to try and talk myself into seeing that my feelings for him weren't legit. That he was my friend. That it was pathetic and silly to pine after a hometown ex I had never even had sex with. How serious could we have been?

IN MY BUDDHISM COURSE, I WAS fascinated by a genre of literature called *namtar*, bringing together two Tibetan words: *nampar*, which means *complete*, and *tharpa*, which means *liberation*. A namtar tells the story of a person's complete liberation from suffering. In a book titled *Women of Wisdom*, Tsultrim Allione explains that these stories "are specifically geared to provide records for those on a spiritual quest, in much the same way that someone about to climb a high mountain would seek out the chronicles of those who had made the climb before." The unifying theme is going to absurd extremes to achieve nirvana.

I expected so-called spiritual quests to be real snoozers, but the stories were hilarious and the women were fierce. They pulled whacky schemes to seek enlightenment back in the day.

An eighteenth-century nun named Orgyan Chokyi fled to a cave to meditate. For Chokyi, solitude did not mean isolation, but separation from gender roles, where she could turn her attention to her mind. She was happiest practicing religious techniques within a community of women. Telling her story, against the orders of her male master, became an expression of freedom.

Another namtar was about a woman whose name was, just to make things confusing, Chokyi Dronma. A fifteenth-century princess, she became pregnant when she was nineteen years old and gave birth to a daughter. During a trip out of town, Dronma's infant died. As the story goes, "This episode gave her much to think about." That was it: *Much to think about.* She expressed that she had no reason to worry since her daughter would be reincarnated. When she was twenty, Dronma longed to give up her royal marriage, just like rich-boy Buddha, and seek enlightenment. After all attempts to persuade her father to let her pursue the dharma—the teachings of Buddha— had failed, she lashed out at her husband, chopping off her hair in a frenzied rage, pretending to have a psychotic episode. It worked. Dronma gave up her royal throne and then persuaded her spiritual masters to ordain her as a monk—a *monk*, not a nun.

Here was a woman who had been pregnant at nineteen, whose only child had died (but would be reincarnated), who pondered the loss deeply but perhaps not too emotionally, and went on to master spiritual law sufficiently enough to become a monk in an order that had historically excluded women. I wasn't trying to dream too big, but I liked the possibilities: reincarnation of a lost baby, a quest for enlightenment, and ordination into a class of masters.

I wanted to be able to write a namtar of my own, a story about my complete liberation from my obsession with motherhood and fixation on marriage and Will-B and Noah and Jade I and Jade II and the layered conspiracy of secrecy and silence about certain aspects of abortion that I felt was forced on me and the mirror of my mother's life. I wanted a namtar about my abortion.

I was accustomed to hearing that religion shackled and chained women, jailed us, oppressed us—and it had, and it did, and it can—but these Tibetan women hadn't escaped from religion; they escaped *to* it. Though they dwelled in a distant time and a faraway place, spiritual practice had torched their shackles and untied their chains.

I was theoretically freed from the bondage these women had to break out of. I didn't have to escape *to* religion in order to escape *from* domestication. I didn't have a baby, though I had been pregnant. I didn't have to marry; lord knew, nobody had deigned to propose to me. I was, for all intents and purposes, available to pursue enlightenment.

"Here's my paper," I said to my Buddhism professor, handing her nineteen stapled pages. My teeth chattered; I was running a fever of 102. My teacher was a tall, willowy scholar with a bright, round face and long black hair that fell down her back like a nun's habit. She asked me what I was working on next.

"Abortion," I wheezed, nonsensically.

"Interesting," she said. Her speech mannerisms were so controlled that she barely moved her mouth. "Have you heard of *mizuko kuyo*?"

"Me-zuke-oo?" I repeated.

"No, meh-zuke-oh kew-yo," she said. "It's a Japanese Buddhist ritual to practice after an abortion." I then experienced a spell of déjà vu that lasted so long I thought it was a side effect of my medicine. It was like I'd just remembered: *that's what I'm supposed to do.* "I might have an article about it somewhere around here," she said, leaning over her file cabinet, flipping through tabs and papers. "Shoot. Seems I can't find the article. Try Google."

"Thank you," I said.

The odds of my professor telling me about an abortion ritual at this precise moment seemed about as high as Noah naming his daughter Jade by pure coincidence. It was such an intense moment of synchronicity that I held the ritual idea like a tiny diamond in my fist. In a mononucleosis haze, I crossed the whirring yellow intersection with a plan that now seems as preposterous as it was prophetic. It was settled in my mind that I would partake of every such healing technique for abortion that I could afford, both religious and secular. My abortion was the heart of my life. A diamond that refracted light into my love partnerships, my friendships, my body, my mind, my ambitions, my beliefs about money, my feelings about womanhood, my relationship with history and with God.

Did rituals and healing techniques exist? That's a question I didn't ask. I was certain they would. I commanded them to.

Going to a holy place to perform a ritual specifically related to abortion would bring me together with other people who wanted to heal after an abortion. We needed a space of our own.

I walked the long hallway to my bedroom, but I didn't Google the rituals. Not yet. Delirious and exhausted, I slept for three weeks. When I woke up, the headline on the front page of the *New York Times* read: "Abortion Doctor Shot to Death in Kansas Church."

IN HIS CHURCH, I THOUGHT, as I boarded a plane hugging my navy blue meditation cushion. I was heading back to Austin to stay with Greg for the summer. I had no plans except to live off my tax returns and make Greg love me. *Shot and killed in his church.*

I so badly wanted to distance myself from slogans of "regret" as-

sociated with the gunman's political party. I so badly did not want
to alienate myself from other people who'd had an abortion if they
weren't asking similar questions or having similar thoughts and feelings. So the next month was a montage of attempts to avoid healing.

I went with friends to watch a movie titled *I Had An Abortion,* which
documents eleven women's stories. One, a punkish girl named Jenny,
talked about hiding the pregnancy and having nobody to talk to. After her abortion, she said she read the Bible, trying to make sense of
what hadn't felt like a baby, but hadn't felt like nothing, either. I almost exploded in tears. Almost. But nobody else in the theater was
losing it, so I focused on the blue veins in my pale hands, which were
shaking in my lap, and turned up my thoughts to a volume that was
louder than the movie. What did I think about? Ice cream. The beach.
Then: the thing that wasn't nothing. My skull throbbed. The room
undulated like it was submerged underwater. The backs of the heads
in front of me morphed into splotches as I subtly gasped for air, stuck
in the middle of a row, having a secret full-blown panic attack.

Next I turned to Greg; I *clung* to Greg, even accompanying him to
the Jewelry Channel studio during his overnight shift. Sometimes I
explored the quiet facility: the padlocked closets storing loose gem-
stones; the framed photographs of engagement rings flanking the
florescent halls, blown-up portraits, diamonds bigger than my head;
bluish-green emeralds, rubies in the jaws of gold princess cuts, glit-
tering bling Will-B might present to Sarah. I felt queasy.

In the doorway of the television studio, I watched Greg, wearing
a black headset, talk to the host. An Eva Menendez doppelganger
in a red shirt, plunging neckline, she slipped rings on and off her
fingers, modeling them for the camera. She and Greg bantered back
and forth, but I couldn't hear what they were saying. Then the host
looked down into her cleavage, adjusted her breasts with both hands.
Her eyes slid up and locked with Greg's. My stomach dropped.

I shifted my gaze, back and forth from Greg to the host, stiff with fear. My thoughts raced. Suddenly it seemed possible to me that he had cheated on me and knocked her up, which made her boobs huge. I tried to pray the crazy away, but what good would a prayer do? I deserved it. They'd buy a house in an area of town populated by newlyweds and name their daughter after a gemstone and I'd end up a lonely idiot.

On the drive home, I gently interrogated Greg about the host's enlarged breasts. He reached across the armrest and took my hand in his, keeping his eyes on the road. "Sorry you're going through that," he said. He turned out to be a master of tai chi boyfriend moves—I'd come at him swinging and there'd be nothing for me to fight against.

With nowhere else to run, I laced up my sneakers and tore off in a dead sprint on a long black road. Temperature pushed 110. No wind, no shade. Then I was light-headed and blacking out. I stopped and crouched down on the scorching asphalt, hugging my knees for I don't know how long, unable to stand up without falling down.

TWO OPTIONS REMAINED: EITHER I STAND in line for paper slippers in a mental hospital or I try to follow the road laid down by enlightened humans—people like Orgyan Chokyi, Chokyi Dronma, Bill Wilson, Jesus, Mary Magdalene, Mother Mary, Buddha, and Dolly Parton.

Greg would pass through his bachelor pad, and there I would be in the den, reading The World's Religions in the plank position. Christianity began when an unwed teen mom carried a baby and gave birth to him in dangerous circumstances, even though she wasn't married and her betrothed wasn't the father. Buddhism began when a man who had everything realized something was missing. He blessed his sleeping wife and son—whom he had named Rahula, which means "fetter," which means shackle—and then departed from his family in search of enlightenment. He set out on a journey through the reli-

gions of his day and then finally sat under the Bodhi tree in meditation and reached his goal. Mary Magdalene had seven demons cast
out and became a spiritual teacher. Bill W. was an alcoholic who went
on to get sober and pen twelve steps prompting drunks to confront
the painful thoughts that made them feel alienated from humanity
without a drink. Dolly Parton grew up getting bullied for being poor,
the inspiration for her transcendent song, "Coat of Many Colors."

Every enlightened master was mercilessly stereotyped and misunderstood. Mary Magdalene: a psychotic whore. Bill: a deadbeat drunk.
Mother Mary: a pregnant teen claiming the father of her child is God.
Buddha: a spoiled trust fund kid with enough money to be poor. Jesus:
a fraudulent guru. Dolly: you get the drift from the bullying she put
up with. The point is, not one of them would have become their utmost
selves by pretending everything was fine or by giving up on their own
story. Once I took my abortion out of the political conflict and put it in
the spiritual realm, a road of healing seemed strangely magical.

"Have you heard of hysteria?" Greg called out to me from his open
bedroom door. I was now doing squats and lunges in his den.

"Are you trying to tell me something?" I hollered back, thrusting my
free weights resolutely into the air, powering through the pangs of fear.
Three weeks after the incident at the Jewelry Channel, I was still nauseated by all the scandalous undressed things I imagined he and the
host could have done together. I said nothing while fear ate my brain.

Greg drew people to him, from elderly people to children, like he
was encased in a magnetic force field. "He reminds you of Will-B," my
mother had said, after they'd met. Greg managed to be both intimate
and emotionally unavailable at the same time, creating worlds and
conspiracies and languages with me, though he was allergic to romance. Our song was Joy Division's "Love Will Tear Us Apart."

Whenever his phone rang, I imagined a woman calling to tell him
he was a father. When I told him about my paranoia, instead of pro-

viding the comfort I expected, he'd say, "This feels like control." I wasn't sure what was worse—actually finding out that he'd strayed, possibly impregnating someone else, or watching with humiliation as he walked out of the room after I'd wrongly accused him of my own mistakes. Today, I was being good. Not asking questions. Just pumping iron and trying not to think.

"No, I'm not trying to tell you anything," Greg said with long Texas vowels. "I somehow ended up on the Wikipedia page for 'hysteria,'" he continued. "Thought you'd find it interesting."

His computer was set up in his lap where he lay in bed in a gray waffle bathrobe. I sidled up to him on the edge of the mattress. I felt a pit in my chest the size of a fist whenever I came into contact with Greg's electronic devices, each potentially possessing evidence of indiscretions. I squinted at the screen: Wikipedia said that the word "hysteria" comes from the Greek word for "womb." Starting around the fourth or fifth century BCE, ancient doctors diagnosed women with this preposterous "illness." When a woman experienced excessive emotion, male physicians believed her womb was traveling around her body. Symptoms purportedly included nervousness, insomnia, faintness, sexual desire *and* loss of sexual desire, heaviness in the abdomen, muscle spasm, shortness of breath, irritability, loss of appetite, and "a tendency to cause trouble."

"'Hysteria stayed on the medical books until 1980,'" Greg read out loud.

"I guess we finally stopped causing trouble," I said, now lying on my back in the yoga pose savasana on the floor. "Until 1980," I repeated, closing my eyes, recalling my research jag from five years earlier when I was pregnant. "The term 'postabortion syndrome' was coined the very next year, in 1981," I told him. "It's basically just an updated term."

I wasn't into conspiracy theories, or maybe I was, but I had noticed that, throughout time, women's minds, wombs, and spiritual gifts had been stigmatized, medicated, subdued, sedated, silenced, taken for granted, and written off. Women had been burned at the stake, stoned to death, drowned, erased from history, sexualized, demonized, and accused of witchcraft. Women had been psychologized, sexualized, and reduced to a label instead of being seen as spiritual powerhouses. So maybe it wasn't a bad sign that strong emotions after abortion had been labeled "postabortion syndrome." Maybe it was just a diversion from the opportunity—in my case, a journey of waking up.

WHEN I BEGAN TO PLAN MY PILGRIMAGE, I had to "work" with cool logic. I carried my laptop out to Greg's fenced-in backyard and sat down on a mound of dirt, leaning against a tree trunk with my computer on my lap, the sun behind the branches striping my legs. It was August, just after my twenty-fifth birthday.

I typed into the Google search field: *abortion ritual healing "not regret" support so many feelings losing my mind HELP.*

I covered the screen with my hands so I wouldn't see any gory pictures posted next to that electric word, but only a log of possibilities shone through my splayed fingers. I flew the arrow of my mouse over the screen, planning for nine months. I worked methodically, as if I were a cartographer drawing a map from abortion to enlightenment.

Father Google showed me the way.

I found three ministrations designed specifically for abortion by practitioners of three major religions: Buddhism (Shin), Christianity (Catholicism), and Judaism (Reconstructionist with a Kabbalistic flair).

Just as my Buddhism professor had told me, there is the Japanese Buddhist ritual *mizuko kuyo*, which was originally for abortion, but which, over time, included miscarriage and stillbirth as well. As I read in William LaFleur's *Liquid Life: Abortion and Buddhism in Japan*, the word *mizuko* means "water baby" or "children of the waters," which I loved. "Fetus" is too medical. "Unborn child" is too political. "Water baby" is just right. Liquid moves from one state to another, from ice to water, water to vapor: solid to invisible.

In Buddhism, we continually grow into our humanness, and we begin leaving this world long before our hearts stop. Instead of entering this planet at birth and exiting at death, we are born and reborn. So the *mizuko* leaves the waters of the womb and returns to an earlier state, with the gods, to a new family, or to the realm of possibilities, the unknown. The same potential child might wait and return to the same parent(s) at a more opportune time. *Kuyo* is simple: it means respect.

Japanese women created the *mizuko kuyo* ritual. Evidence suggests that the rite began in the 1600s. Japan had virtually no public debate about reproductive rights. This blew me away. Picketers didn't line up outside clinics. Doctors weren't gunned down in their places of worship. I could hardly imagine growing up in a country without an abortion war. There was a brief kerfuffle when *mabiki*—the Japanese word for thinning or pruning in a garden that is used metaphorically to refer to abortion—was banned from 1868 to 1948 because the population was in decline. The government portrayed motherhood as a patriotic duty and distributed tablets depicting women who chose *mabiki* as having devil horns. Women continued to end their pregnancies secretly and still performed the ritual. The ritual was their choice. I wanted to replace the conflict in my imagination with an alternative: a peaceful and empowering vision of mourning.

I phoned twelve Buddhist temples and centers and churches in all five boroughs of New York City. Reverend T.K. returned my call from a church ten blocks away from my apartment.

"Can you bring a photograph of the water baby?" he asked, trebling with a Japanese accent. A *photograph?* Was this a test?

"I didn't ask for a picture at Planned Parenthood," I said, hoping he would get the hint.

"Oh. I see," he'd said, with a nervous laugh. "Just bring a flower then." We scheduled the ritual—my very first—for March.

Next was Christianity. Wow: Jesus never mentioned the word *abortion,* even though it was practiced during his time on earth.

In Roman Catholicism, an American psychologist named Theresa Burke designed a ministry for healing after abortion. In 1994, she organized a weekend of theatrical rituals aimed to help cleanse people like me of fear, shame, and numbness.

The retreat is called Rachel's Vineyard. "Individuals of all denominations are welcome," a brochure reads. I assumed this meant that my personal religion—a speedball teaching of the Twelve Steps, Buddha, Jesus, Mary Magdalene, and Dolly Parton—would be welcome. A blurb from an alumna assured me I'd fit right in: "I hesitated to come because I knew it would be intense and I wasn't 100 percent committed to the religious concepts (or I was leery of them). The retreat far surpassed my expectations." Hoping to feel a shred more peaceful, I decided to attend and mailed a $100 check to Rachel's Vineyard to sign up for the next session.

Then I dashed off an email to Rabbi Rayzel Raphael, who conceived the first recorded Jewish ritual for abortion in the United States. Her tie-dye psychedelic website describes her as "unorthodox, creative, fun, feminist, lighthearted, funny, wise." She emailed me her spiritual autobiography, which showed me that I wouldn't have to explain my despair to her. She had been there. I caught her on her cell phone between appointments near her home in Pennsylvania.

"You've been carrying this for a while." She had a smoky southern accent. "Pen a letter to the soul that you sent on in a different direction and then get back to me."

I liked her style—I responded well to a businesslike approach to healing.

Then there were Hindu practitioners. Hindu culture and practice have rituals for everything. They have rituals for their rituals. One for conception. Another for protection. A ritual for the cravings of a pregnant woman. For birth. Longevity. Naming. Y'all, they have a ritual for taking a child outdoors for the first time, and yet another for its first bite of solid food. But there was neither a bell for me to ring nor a vow to recite nor a single god for me to petition in the entire polytheistic herd of more than thirty million gods. I found this hard to believe. India, where Hinduism began, legalized abortion in 1971, two years before the United States.

I emailed Professor Douglas R. Brooks, a leading scholar of Hinduism, at University of Rochester, to sleuth for some insider information. He replied: "Abortion has been practiced in India as long as there have been human beings, but there is, to my knowledge, no sanction or process of acknowledgment that is part of the ritual traditions. You're not likely to find what you are looking for except in the pages of anthropological research."

I checked the pages of anthropological research and didn't come across a ritual there, either. Though I did find a relevant quotation in the sacred text *Hymns of the Atharva-Veda,* under the heading "Expiation for certain heinous crimes": "Enter into the rays, into smoke, O sin; go into the vapours, and into the fog! Lose thyself on the foam of the river! Wipe off, O Pushan, the misdeeds upon him that practiseth abortion!" I could only hope that when this quest was over, my "sin" would vanish.

I scrolled through websites and read books about Islam. The Qur'an does not mention abortion. From what I could tell, each school of Islam established their own rules about ending a pregnancy. One set of instructions in Islam was to practice the "ABC [*sic*] of Repentance":

A. "You must admit the guilt." (Check-ish, though the Catholics would help me to tease that out.)

B. "Deep down in your heart, you feel sorry for your mistake." (Check—for the mistake of getting pregnant by accident.)

C. "You must enter into a sincere covenant with your Lord that you have totally closed those dark pages, and you will never open them again." (Yikes—I was about to open those dark pages.)

So I was still learning my ABC of Repentance.

By the time my search expanded, I was back in Manhattan in a new apartment building, directly across the street from my first one. Greg sat reading a book on the love seat in the other room, before he had to skedaddle for his shift at a new production company. I sat in my closet-cum-office and typed in the blue square of my computer screen light, continuing to plan my pilgrimage.

California had cornered the secular market on postabortion healing rituals: Ava Torre-Bueno was a veteran Planned Parenthood counselor who risked her reputation during training sessions with pro-choice activists by leading an exercise that played into anti-choice arguments: she asked them to choose a loss to mourn and then handed out long pieces of fabric that made a visceral masking tape sound when torn. Ripping the fabric brought the activists to tears. Terrified of grief and everything I thought it meant about my pregnancy, I wanted Ava to tell me that my problems could be solved by any other means possible. I didn't know how to grieve without losing the ability to function. I definitely didn't know where grief was located on the path of enlightenment.

Terra Wise, also known as the "Midwife for the Soul," specialized in helping people like me birth new parts of the self, a process she coined "Womb Wisdom."

The social scientist Kate Cockrill had conducted a study of emotions around abortion, a territory that few scholars had dared to navigate; she interviewed hundreds of women about their experiences. I hoped she would assure me that other people felt similarly. I wanted confirmation that feminists I loved wouldn't think of me as a turncoat if I talked about my abortion without fronting—that I'd keep my seat in the club.

Aspen Baker, the executive director of the nation's only apolitical abortion hotline, had listened to thousands of men and women over the phone, recognizing that the pro-life/pro-choice conflict had hidden the real conversations happening behind the scenes. Inspired by her callers, she started a peace movement to end the abortion war that she called pro-voice, and that's what drew me to her: the possibility of a collective of people who met face-to-face.

Among my godless friends and stoical Protestant kin, I disguised my pilgrimage as intellectual inquiry.

"I'm going on a research trip to California," I said to my mother during our daily phone call. I could hear her blending a SlimFast shake in her new husband's kitchen. I'd planned on shooting out to the West Coast alone with the Indigo Girls in the tape deck and a trusty box of tissues in the passenger's seat, but Mom insisted that I invite a travel companion: her.

"I don't want you driving all over California by yourself," she said.

"Mom. I'll be fine."

"You buy your own plane ticket to California, but I'll book the hotels," she said, "You hear?"

"I hear."

"You find us a car to drive," she said. "From a real car place, okay? And a fun car. I'm retired and remarried. I get to drive fun cars these days."

"You got it," I told her.

She would finance a more reliable ride than a vehicle from Rent-A-Wreck and more plush sleeping arrangements than the hostels in which I had planned to bunk along the coastline.

The journey would begin at the *mizuko kuyo* ritual at a Buddhist Church. Then I'd ride a train to Long Island for Rachel's Vineyard, the retreat inspired by Roman Catholicism. Next, I'd fly to California to meet my mom. Our road trip would follow Highway 1.

"Sounds like an adventure," she said.

So it began, my three-year journey. I didn't know what it meant to "birth new parts of myself." I didn't feel particularly guilty, at least not in the traditional sense of the word. I didn't know how a Roman Catholic retreat could fix my paranoid suspicions about Greg. I just knew that recovering after abortion had to contain more depth and substance than hearing, "You made the right decision." Or: "You are not alone," a slogan that rang hollow when so many of us felt alone—without a place to express ourselves completely. If I had mistakes to correct, then denying them would make me feel unresolved, or even defensive. But I wanted to be forgiven without being pushed to ask for forgiveness. I wanted to confront my decision to have an abortion with clarity; but I wasn't going to let anyone poach my thoughts and emotions for a political agenda. The rule was self-compassion. The goal was enlightenment.

II.
ABORTION
RITES
FOR
BETTER
LIVING

MY APOLOGY

SIX YEARS AFTERWARD— On a bright morning in March, I headed toward the New York Buddhist Church with a broken brain and a sticky note in my back pocket. The note read: RITUAL AT 11 A.M. RING ALL FOUR DOORBELLS. Trees in the medians had turned pink and white, thousands of petals fluttering and swirling down and landing on my crochet sweater like snowfall. I wove through the crowded sidewalk, past two Indian teenagers holding hands on a bench, past an elderly white woman with a long blue braid and an armful of books, past an Asian businessman talking into a tiny cell phone and pushing a baby carriage. I thought of how strange and estranged we all are, that I could be en route to an abortion ritual, that anyone I see, at any given time, could be in the midst of anything serious at all.

I stopped at a bodega to pick out a bouquet of blue irises for the reverend—my monk friend Ernie told me to bring him a gift—as well as a flower for the water baby, per Reverend T.K.'s instructions. I wasn't sure what kind of flower dust in the ether would want, but my eyes landed on a bucket of daisies. One seemed to be reaching for me. The petals were yellow and stitched with tangerine, radiating around a red disk. I plucked it out by the stem, feeling sad about my fragile daisy. Noah had a baby. I had a flower. Baby. Flower. I handed the bearded clerk a couple of crumpled dollar bills, thinking, *If only you knew.*

After a five-minute walk down the sidewalk, I looked up at a statue of a man named Shinran Shonin, the founder of the Jodo Shinshu School, or Shin Buddhism, at the entrance of the New York Buddhist Church. The statue had survived the atomic bomb before it was transported to my neighborhood of Manhattan. He was fifteen feet tall, donning a conical sun hat and holding a staff in his hand. I'd researched him, too. Shinran Shonin learned to recognize all beings as Buddha in disguise, and all people as awakened. Buddha comes to earth to teach lessons dressed up as everyone we meet: my mother, my exes, my water baby.

I stood at the door of my first ritual. The door of no return. Because when you start any process of healing, even if you make a humble beginning, there's no turning back. You're in, even if you're trying not to be. And it was one thing to engage in a private brawl with my conscience, but it was quite another to stand before a Buddhist priest and profess that I turned my baby away and, six years later, was still not quite over it. Part of me wished I could step back in time to seventeenth-century Japan, a gathering on the crossroads.

I rang all four bells.

While I waited, I recalled last night's nightmare. Another nightmare. The hundredth nightmare of what had started to feel like the only baby, never born: I'd lost my baby at a house party, but I couldn't admit to anyone that I had a baby, so I couldn't ask anyone for help finding her. I searched for her on my hands and knees, cigarette smoke in my eyes, opening closet doors and checking the bathtub. In the kitchen, a crowd of college students parted like a curtain to reveal my baby lying on the counter like a moldy loaf of bread. I took her cold body into my arms. Next I was riding down a highway, engine roaring, shadows rolling over the windshield like ghosts. My mother was with me, but nobody in particular was driving. The baby was in the trunk. We pulled up in front of an emergency room and I put her on the sidewalk near the glass entrance.

Inside the Buddhist church, I would look for a small stone statue of Jizo, the bodhisattva of departed children, fertility, and cross-roads. Bodhisattvas are gods and goddesses who stopped short of reaching full-blown Buddhahood. Their pre-Buddha status allows them to identify with everyday human suffering and lead humans to enlightenment, somewhat analogous to Jesus Christ. A bodhi-sattva shows absolute compassion. The bodhisattva Jizo is said to understand why a person would have an abortion. He blesses future children. He blesses crossroads—decisive moments—and travelers. In Japan, statues of Jizo stand guard at intersections. This was the start of my pilgrimage, and I liked to think that he'd watch over the rest of it.

Jizo was there for the water babies, too. He'd steer the little one through the dark realms of the afterlife to ensure a high rebirth. In certain sects of Buddhism, an aborted being is believed to have bad karma from a previous incarnation. The abortion would be consid-ered its punishment, but Jizo corrects a water baby's karma.

Some Buddhist temples in Japan are dedicated solely to *mizuko kuyo*, one with more than fifty thousand gray Jizo statues in red bibs packing the grassy knolls, each figure illustrating a specific loss and personalized with family names, like tombstones. Although some such temples have been perceived as controversial money-making endeavors, it isn't unusual for Japanese to pay respects to Jizos regu-larly, just as I visited my grandmothers' and friends' graves, leaving flowers and notes. Parents take their living children to the Jizos as a way of "introducing" them to their late sibling, even "inviting" them to movie night. In Japan, writes memoirist Marie Mutsuki Mockett, "the dead miss us as much as we miss them." I could only imagine how a tombstone for a water baby would go over with my hilarious girlfriends and hyperrational mother, but secretly, I loved it. I loved the idea that the dead joined the living, that ancestors, young and old, were remembered.

In the seventeenth century, when *mizuko kuyo* rituals began, the most common abortion a doctor prescribed was a mercury brew that a woman could drink to end a pregnancy—and those who couldn't afford a doctor would resort to more brutal techniques. Then she could meet "the cult of Jizo," as the gathering was known, on the roadside—at "the crossroads"—and participate in the first version of the ritual. I imagined women gathering to wash stone statues the color of slate and praying that the bodhisattva Jizo would lead their water babies in a parade through the underworld. I loved how a Japanese woman had a place to go after an abortion, how women banded together in public, how they thanked their compassionate god and their water babies.

Back in the twenty-first century, at the New York Buddhist Church, a barefoot man positioned himself snug in the doorframe. He was wearing a karate uniform, a black belt secured at his dense middle. He puffed out his chest.

"Is the reverend expecting you?" He sounded like the Fonz.

"We have an appointment at 11," I said.

He watched me for two beats. I pictured the Fonz in a karate uniform.

"So you have an appointment? And he's expecting you?"

"Yes and yes."

It was my outfit: skinny jeans and brown cowgirl boots that looked like I found them in a Dumpster. Had to be my outfit. I explained that I was there for the ritual, but not what kind. I assumed other people would be in attendance, which was typical in Japan. I held up the bouquet of blue irises. "For the reverend," I said.

He invited me into the foyer.

"Wait here," he said, pointing to a couch. "I'll call T.K."

The Fonz bounded down a flight of steps into what I assumed was the basement. I studied the mantel across the room. Gold statues of Laughing Buddhas with big bellies. A white sign leaned against a wall with this Japanese character: 道. And the translation below: "PATH."

At 11:47 A.M., there was still no sign of the reverend.

I could hear grunting from the basement: "Huh. HUH. HUH."

I decided my best bet was to make noises to remind the karate priest that I was up here. I stomped back and forth across the foyer. I rapped on a wall. I traipsed down the staircase to a landing and kicked a step. If there were pots and pans, I would have banged them.

"HUH. HUH."

I ventured down two more steps. One of the four doorbells I had rung had been labeled "bedroom." The karate priest had given me stern instructions to wait on the couch.

"EXCUSE ME," I called, but there was no answer. I had been planning this rite of passage for nearly a year. It had taken all the courage I had to walk over the threshold of my first ritual. I had nightmares. Nausea. A flower for my water baby. And nobody was here to meet me.

Waiting: a tragicomic metaphor for asking a person to wait to be born.

In the basement, I walked through a dim hallway. The groaning and wheezing grew louder. I found an open door and pressed my back flat against the wall, for fear it was the bedroom. I bent forward to look through the doorway and then snapped back into place. It wasn't a bedroom. It was a gymnasium.

The Fonz poked his head out of the door. His black hair was slicked straight up.

"Hey," he said, cocking his chin. "T.K. didn't answer his cell. Not sure where he is. His Honda's here."

We went back upstairs together and stood chatting in the foyer. This guy wasn't a Buddhist priest, after all—just the building manager in a karate uniform.

"May I leave a note?" I asked. "We were supposed to do that ritual."

"Did somebody die?"

"Sort of," I replied, not quite sure what I believed.

"I GOT STOOD UP BY A PRIEST," I said to Greg. I found him reading a Solzhenitsyn paperback at our long wood table. "I bet he's just out rescuing sentient beings," he said. I pecked him on the cheek as I floated past and locked myself in the bedroom.

There was the bed, the altar of my nightmares. I took my pillow and clutched it with both hands, trying to tear it apart—as if that would destroy my subconscious activity, my mind. In another terror from last night, I was teaching a class and remembered that I'd left a baby at home alone, so I ran through campus, trying to get back to the baby. Students stopped me and asked me to grade their papers. Friends rushed up to me in tears. I felt like my mother when she left me to wait for her on the front steps of my closed high school until dark when I was a freshman. "I'm sorry," I said out loud, wondering where that came from.

One purpose of the *mizuko kuyo* ritual is to apologize.

In the nightmare, I feared I would return home to a dead baby. Instead, Greg had the toddler set up cooing in her playpen, and he was serving her a bowl of colorful vegetables, so bright they looked fake. Then I woke up and remembered what had really happened—that I'd had an invaded womb and a confused boyfriend. I thought of Noah's Jade. "I'm sorry," I said again.

The ritual had begun.

I had heard well-meaning women tell one another under the guise of empowerment to stop saying the word "sorry." But I had a *Sorry* inside of me that needed to come out. During the *mizuko kuyo* ritual, the apology was an act of respect and gratitude toward the potential child. *I'm sorry I couldn't bring you to the planet at that time, but thank you for waiting for a better time (and possibly for a different parent).*

I used to brace myself never to apologize for my abortion, protecting my *Sorry* against anyone who might try to capture it and put it in a jar and bring it to the Sorry Laboratory to pick apart and misinterpret. But this apology was mine.

We don't apologize just to be forgiven. We apologize to forgive ourselves.

I sorried at the top of my lungs. *I'M SORRY. I. AM. SORRY.*

Holding the pillow with both hands, I told the water baby precisely why I was sorry, hitting the bed for each and every reason. *This one's for disassociating and white-knuckling the procedure,* I thought. *This one's for bad sex education. For untreated addiction. For shoddy self-esteem. For not trusting myself.*

Sorry that my "choices" seemed so awful: either drop out of college and move back home to hide out, or terminate. Sorry I felt so alone. Sorry that I didn't know I could keep the baby, my independence, and my education in Vermont all at the same time. Sorry my world wasn't set up for all three. This one's for thinking I had to become an idealized version of myself, with a swank master's degree and a fancy job title and a standup husband before I'd be good enough for motherhood, for setting myself up to strive to become a perfect future self, but then never feeling I've become her.

I was sorry about the abortion, not necessarily because I'd made the wrong choice, but because other voices had been so loud that I hadn't been able to hear my own. Nineteen years of listening to the schizophrenic collective conscience about girls and pregnant people and motherhood and money had filled my head with opinions that did not belong to me.

This one's for not being able to make the choice in peace.

One hopes to avoid an unwanted pregnancy altogether, but I loved my embryo. It didn't feel right to apologize for creating it. I wasn't sorry about that.

I dropped the pillow on the bed like I was dropping a microphone and opened the bedroom door. Shit. Greg was standing there.

"Tell me you didn't hear that," I said.

"You've got a call," he said, holding up my cell phone.

"Hello?"

It was the Fonz. "Reverend T.K. is ready for you now."

THE WROUGHT-IRON DOOR TO THE CHURCH yawned open and there stood Reverend T.K. in his black robes, flashing me a repentant grin of straight, white teeth. His light brown head was bald as an egg. Black eyebrows hung down into his lids like mini-comb-overs.

"I'm so sorry," he whispered, inviting me into the familiar foyer. He was younger than he sounded over the phone. Mid-thirties. I'd never allowed myself to crush on a priest, but he was a bit of a dreamboat. I pictured him in jeans, a plain white T-shirt, and for some reason, smoking a cigarette. Like a Japanese James Dean.

"These are for you." I handed him the sprawling bouquet of blue irises, keeping the water baby's daisy for the ritual. Cradling the flowers in his arm, he jogged into the innards of the building, his layered robes flapping out of sight. Bamboo flute music filled the foyer with hollow vibrations that curled around my ears. I had a pebble in my throat, but I wasn't going to break down in front of a Buddhist priest I had just met, crying about someone I'd never meet.

I followed Reverend T.K. through a doorway into the church's Buddha Hall, a cavernous chapel that burst with reds, golds, and purples. The Buddha Hall was so magnificent and decadent, the air jammed in my lungs. Nothing could have prepared me for the beauty of this room or the sadness infused in it. We walked down the center aisle, a long red carpet rolled out for an invisible star. Candlesticks flanked the altar with teardrop flames. A vase of soaring flowers put my wilted daisy to shame.

A huge gold cage was suspended over the altar; it was larger than a dog's crate, about the size of a go-go dancer's cage. A life-size statue of Amitābha, the Buddha of Boundless Love and Boundless Light, sat cross-legged inside.

"Is Jizo here?" I asked.

Reverend T.K. pointed to the statue of Jizo on the red-carpeted platform. Jizo was about a foot tall and colored a dark shade of slate. He clasped his small hands together. His face was frozen into a simple smile. He wore a robe, which made him look like a king baby.

Abortion is diffuseness. It is everywhere and it is nowhere. Jizo represented a loss that I couldn't see—I hadn't even looked at the ultrasound monitor.

The blue irises drooped over a glass vase on the floor. Reverend T.K. probably couldn't fathom that I had brought him a whole bouquet but had brought the embryo child I had aborted only a single daisy.

I sat anxiously in the front row with my hands folded, the daisy laid across my lap.

"So, basically," Reverend T.K. began, "I chant. We meditate. We think of happy wishes for the well-being of the water baby." He cooed *water baby* like it was one word, as if it were a new species. "Please sit up straight and we will do a meditation."

He installed himself behind a sturdy wooden desk and began pounding a gong with his knuckles. Its wobbly reverberations bounced up the walls, fell down to the tops of the chairs and onto Jizo's head. Reverend T.K. moaned into the mic on his desk. *Namu Amida Butsu,* he chanted. *Naaaaaa-mmmmuuuu Amm-eeeeeeee-daaaaaaaa Buuuuuuuuu-t!-suuuuuuu.*

Hail to Amitābha Buddha.

Rising from his seat, he paced back and forth across the platform with long, haunting steps, his black robe lifting like wings. I was nearly levitating off my chair in anticipation. He pressed his hands together and bowed to a bowl of incense. To the candle flames. To the flowers. I was waiting for something major to happen, something like my baby lowering down from the ceiling in a puff of smoke.

"Chant with me," he said, holding up a sutra that was bound with soft purple leather. The top half of the page was scrawled with Japanese characters, accompanied by phonetic capitalized letters. The bottom half had an English translation.

"These words?" I pointed to the English translation.

He nodded absently, seated again behind his desk.

The reverend tucked his chin into his chest, droning into the microphone's fuzz. He banged the giant gong beside him. I watched him intently, almost glaring, trying to determine what he wanted me to do. He bulged his eyes at me, as if to say, "Anytime now." I stared back at him, waiting for him to stop making those noises and start reading the English words.

Instead, he stopped chanting altogether.

My eyes slid up to the phonetic Japanese at the top of the page, the words he had been chanting all along. I began mouthing every fifth syllable on the page, puckering my lips into Os and straining my lips into mute Es, but the choreography was off. I had missed my cue.

I had botched the ritual.

Coming to my rescue, Reverend T.K. took off in a freestyle chant by himself and started walking slowly to the front of the stage, looking at me and moaning like it was nothing. Without breaking eye contact, he beckoned me to the altar, instructing me to make an offering to the water baby and to Jizo as well. I must have approached the altar too casually, because he pressed his hands together emphatically, repeatedly clasping and unclasping them to indicate the appropriate gesture. I sandwiched my hands together and met him with my back stiff like a kid getting measured at the doctor's office. We were squared up, two feet apart.

"The left hand is seen as defiled, unclean," he said, giving me a dharma talk, a teaching, like a sermon. "The right hand is good, light, enlightenment. When we clasp them together, we take good and bad together. Sometimes life isn't wonderful, but we keep going. We don't know if life will be very short, such as your water baby's, or very long, one hundred years. So we must live in this very moment and have compassion for all living things."

He angled a dish of loose red incense toward me. I tossed a pinch of it into a smoldering bowl. It produced a smoky sweet aroma. I turned to the smiling Jizo and did something I had never done before. I bowed, like my water baby was royalty. Buddha in disguise.

My overwhelming question had been, Is the water baby okay? Reborn to another parent? Departed, never having been a thing?

Part of me said, *It never existed.*

A second part said, *Of course it's not okay. It will never be okay.*

A third part said, *You have to keep going.* This was the quietest part.

I came closer to Reverend T.K., close enough to notice that he smelled like the incense coiling up from the altar. He dipped his finger in oil and touched my forehead three times. His fingertip felt hot. Each dab represented one of the Three Jewels: once for the Buddha (the Awakened One), once for the dharma (the teachings), and once for the *sangha* (the community).

He turned around with a flip of his robes and crouched behind the podium. Then he popped back up and loped down to the front of the platform, carrying a long, thin strip of paper, and handed it to me. I stretched out the scroll, end to end, and looked at it. Japanese characters brushed down the ream in feathery black watercolor, spelling the name Amitābha.

"Use this paper," said the reverend. "Say little prayers to it to remind you of the water baby. Wish for its well-being."

"Thank you," I said.

But I didn't want to think about my abortion. I never did. But I had thought of it anyway. Left unattended, my emotional disturbances never really "went away"—they just threw on new costumes and showed up as anger, depression, and nightmares. To stop remembering against my will, I would have to remember intentionally. It was important to note that "remembrance" did not mean weeping in bed for twelve hours, writhing in mental agony, and eating a box of Oreos while watching *The Bachelor* without any pants on.

The act of remembrance had instructions in its Latin root: *rememorari*. *Re* means "again"; *memorari* means "be mindful of." Be mindful, again, and again, and again.

To follow Reverend T.K.'s directions, I would have to revise the way I remembered. The aborted ball of light was helping to wake me up. The water baby was my Buddha.

Reverend T.K. unclasped his hands. I unclasped mine. We ambled back up the red carpet.

"How'd you know about *mizuko kuyo*?" he asked.

"I had a *mabiki*," I said, sure I was misusing the word. "Why?" Why else would I have come?

"Not many Americans know about it."

He told me that Japanese members of his congregation requested the ritual from time to time, but more often, they offered incense during a regular church service without indicating to whom they were dedicating the pinch, since they didn't want anyone to know about their *mizukos*.

"Was this a ritual specifically for the water baby?" I asked.

"No," he said. The ritual had been nothing more than a memorial service.

"Was there anything about this ritual particular to a *mizuko*?"

"I put Jizo over there on the carpet, but the *mizuko* is equal to any other ancestor," said Reverend T.K. "It doesn't need a special ritual. Oh, but I usually give the *mizuko* a dharma name. It's nice to have a name. You can remember better with a name."

"What would my *mizuko's* name be?" I asked.

"Hmm . . ." He released a nervous laugh. "Well, it would be kinda weird now. Ritual's over."

"It's okay if it's kinda weird," I said.

"Hmm . . . ," he said again. "The name is *Shaku*."

"I love it!"

"Well, every name has *Shaku* in it. It comes from *Shakyamuni*. It means a disciple of the Buddha."

"I still like it," I said. We giggled. Then he paused for what felt like ten minutes.

"The name of your *mizuko kuyō* is *Shaku Dōkō*," he said at last. I braced myself for the meaning in English, afraid it would make me sadder. Actually, the name was perfect. "*Dōkō* means Guiding Light," said Reverend T.K.

Guiding Light.

"'*Dō*' (導) means 'to guide,'" Reverend T.K. explained. "It consists of the words 'path' (道) and 'inch' (寸). We make one inch of progress at a time. '*Kō*' (光) means 'light.' Light represents many things: light of compassion, light of wisdom, light of truth."

"*Shaku Doko*," I said, rhyming *Dōkō* with Dodo.

"Oh, no," said Reverend T.K. "It's pronounced more like '*deeookō*.'"

"*Shaku Deeookō*," I said.

"The *mizuko* is your guide on the path to enlightenment," he said.

"Thank you."

I headed back to the street, as though there were nothing extraordinary about this day, when in fact, this day had been quite extraordinary. Because it was the first day I had walked up to a door with promises of healing behind it, rung four doorbells, gone in, waited an hour, left, come back, done a ritual, botched the ritual, found out it wasn't the ritual I thought it was, and then went on my merry way with a little bit of light, satisfied because I had tried.

I walked along the cobblestone path, past the people on park benches, the woman reading a newspaper, the man playing a saxophone that honked in spurts. I carried the strip of paper in my hand, letting it flutter in the wind like a flag.

In my office, I pushed a tack through the top of my flag for Guiding Light, hanging it down the side of the window.

A miracle happened that night: I did not dream of the baby. Not that night. Not the next night or the night after that.

The nightmares had stopped.

SUSPICIOUS MINDS

SIX YEARS, ONE MONTH, AND TWO WEEKS AFTERWARD — I stuffed pants and shirts into my burnt orange duffle bag, trying not to think about all the women I was sure Greg would bring to the apartment on my first trip away from him. The novelist in the cardigan sweater who looked like his mother: fragile bones, quiet, focused. Or someone I'd never met before, maybe a co-worker from his television production job in Connecticut.

Everybody was a suspect. Receipts had become "evidence." Even the mailbox seemed liable to contain confirmation of a transgression, though the most recent letter was a thick envelope from Rachel's Vineyard, the Roman Catholic retreat I'd signed up for. Expecting it to contain an itinerary of the weekend, I eagerly tore it open and pulled out a glossy card, embossed with a sleeping black baby, chubby wrists looking like loaves of bread.

A thank-you note for a donation?

Vince, a deacon in the church, apologized via email. My check had fallen into the wrong pile. I had told him I was vegan and asked whether I should bring my own stash of food to the retreat. Vince shooed me off: "We have you covered with your veganism." He instructed me to take a train from Penn Station to a town on the north shore of Long Island. He would dispatch one of his brethren to pick me up.

I expected all political persuasions to be left at the door. I couldn't fathom a place for healing after abortion that openly condemned it. I was convinced the retreat would lean toward the Catholics for Choice school of thought, a movement that, according to the organization's website, "supports a woman's moral and legal right to follow her conscience in matters of sexuality and reproductive health."

I grabbed my cell phone charger and tossed it in my bag, then stood before my jewelry rack to select a couple of necklaces to pack, trying to power through my paranoid thoughts of what could happen in this bedroom, our bed, this weekend.

MY BRAIN STILL FELT BROKEN. Back in Austin, before the move to New York, I had started asking Greg to account for each millisecond of his day, justify his whereabouts, leave no idle moment unexplained. I knew how quickly a slip could happen: one minute, you're walking toward the bathroom in the dorms, and the next, you've got a water baby.

"How was lunch with Clete?" I had asked him.

"Good," he'd said absently, stirring his coffee with a spoon. "He says hi."

"Aw, I love Clete," I'd gushed. And I did love Clete, but then I'd build the conversation, block by block, asking who else dined with them, what time he had arrived at the restaurant, how long they stayed, where he went next, and what time it was as he was driving away from the restaurant, all while reading his nonverbal cues for signs of deception.

"We're not having the same conversation, are we," he'd said, noticing that I was calculating time frames and distances. "You're gathering evidence to bust me in an affair." I tried to strengthen the muscle of trust by withholding my questions and going to the bathroom to pray on my knees instead, but some thoughts wouldn't go away. I hoped he could make me believe him, but instead he'd repeated his mantra: "I can't fix this."

Then, we'd set out to drive 1,743 miles from Austin to Upper Manhattan in a rental car packed with his boxes. Somewhere around Memphis, I cracked. I couldn't stop thinking about a name I had accidentally glimpsed in his inbox. The name matched his ex-wife's.

"I saw an email from Jennifer in your inbox," I confessed with an even tone of voice, hugging my stomach, needing his assurance, yet knowing that no matter how he answered the question, I would find him guilty. It was midnight. Headlights floated toward and past us. The anticipation of hearing him tell me he'd had sex with someone else was maddening, sickening, intoxicating. Sometimes I wished he would just get it over with and prove me right. Sometimes I worried that if he hadn't cheated on me yet, I'd drive him to it now.

"Man, what the f*ck," said Greg. "Jennifer is the accounts payable clerk from the Jewelry Channel. Not my wife," he said. *Ex*-wife, I thought.

"Sorry," I responded, combing my fingers through my cutoffs. "I'm trying."

"I just sold my car, quit my job, and left my friends and family for you. Try harder."

He veered onto an exit ramp and sped down a lightless road, two headlamps in the fog. A red blur glowed in the distance. I hugged my knees to my chest in the passenger's seat, as the hazy red light became a gas station sign.

"I hate it as much as you do," I told him. "Intellectually, I know I'm probably just projecting onto you my guilt about my own past indiscretions"—*or was I?*—"but I can't stop thinking that you'll cheat on me." He parked under the lights without speaking. So I continued. "Right now, my brain tells me that when I asked you about Jennifer, you told the truth on a technicality, and really opened a secret email account to have an affair with someone who isn't named Jennifer." I braced myself for his answer, in case I'd caught him this time, but he threw open the car door and got out, slamming the door behind him. Then he stuck his head through the open window.

"I accused my wife of having affairs. Constantly. She never cheated on me, but I annihilated our marriage within six months. I left. She didn't. Do you get it?"

I got it: every time I accused Greg, I dredged up the marriage he had destroyed with allegations of cheating. Every time I looked at him, I saw the relationship I had destroyed by cheating, the water baby I didn't have. In either role—accuser or cheater—I was the destroyer of love.

By the time we moved up north, he had lost sympathy and refused to comfort me.

Suspicion became my master. I couldn't even watch films or read books about infidelity, which eliminated *Fear of Flying* from my rotation of favorite novels.

I watched my girlfriends go insane with jealousy but then get better. One tracked down her estranged father and proved to herself that he and her doting husband were two different people—and the fixation ended. Another prayed for the happiness of her mate when she felt tempted to probe him (her prayers must have been more potent than mine). Another's photographer fiancé explained that it was his job to capture beauty and invited her on his shoots. I prayed for Greg, meditated on trust, inventoried my fears, withheld my questions. But I only got worse. Now I practiced "controlled suspicion," meaning I didn't bring up my concerns until I lost the ability to function.

But I had made progress at the Buddhist ritual. Acknowledging the *mizuko* in front of a priest had banished my nightmares. The water baby had returned to an earlier state.

I finally felt like I was moving forward. Rachel's Vineyard would bring together a group of people like me, who could speak my language, people who would understand each other implicitly, enlightenment-seeking "cronies," as my dad would say.

I wanted to be forgiven without feeling obligated to want forgiveness. I wanted to forgive other people, too. Forgiving Noah seemed possible. Forgiving myself seemed imperative.

I also wanted to forgive the seemingly unforgiveable. The shooters, bombers, and arsonists against reproductive freedom. The priests and pastors tacitly encouraging the violence. Abortion clinic protesters. Anti-choice billboard funders. I figured the leaders of Rachel's Vineyard must have forgiven these people. They might even share a church pew with some of them on Sunday mornings.

GREG BURST INTO THE ROOM AND sat down on the bed in front of me while I zipped up my bag. "My dad doesn't think you should go," he said. Greg's short hair curled around the sides of his ears like a 1960s rocker. A few gray strands were the only signs of his thirty-eight years. Otherwise, he looked boyish and rugged in a thin T-shirt.

Greg's father, a trial lawyer, was the type of man who'd take us out to a five-star restaurant in bedroom slippers, eat fast, and then drive home separately. Greg was the type of man who preferred meat but ate three vegan meals a day just so he and I could bond over the same cuisine.

"Why shouldn't I go?" I asked, spraying Chanel on my wrists and rubbing them together in front of the round vanity mirror. Even a new mannerism of his could trigger a paranoia attack: *Where'd he learn to move his arm like that?* Every word he said, I could distort into evidence of infidelity. I vacillated between watching him intently and trying not to look at him at all.

"Dad thinks this place could be abusive," Greg said. "They might use the authority of the church and cause psychological damage. I'm saying they could pull some weird-ass shit."

I'd always heard about the Catholic Church's remarkable track record for shaming people under the guise of helping. Take Mary Magdalene. Ever since I could remember, I thought she was a prostitute. I was deeply disappointed to learn that she wasn't. She was a student of Jesus—some say the word "companion" is more accurate—and a spiritual leader. Her name had been raked through the mind of a sixth-century pope who'd portrayed her as a prostitute in a sermon. Once upon a time, the word "prostitute" included unmarried pregnant females. In Ireland, abortion was (and is) illegal. With no choice but to carry to term, unwed mothers were separated from their newborns and imprisoned, forced to wash clothes in grueling laundries, often as a method of "reform," all in the name of my biblical heroine. They were girls like me, considered a stain on Irish Catholic society and sinful beyond reform. Many died in these "asylums." The last Magdalene Laundry closed down in October 1996. Eight years later, I was pregnant. A "prostitute" by some old standards.

Roman Catholics got a bad rap for imposing guilt, but, to their credit, they also understood the psychological value of admitting to a wrong. I didn't like to think of myself as a guilty person, but guilt is normal, and it's hell, but once a wrong is admitted and corrected, voila! The guilt is gone. Being free means being free of guilt. I'd be able to tell the difference between culturally constructed guilt and natural transformative guilt. No need to walk into the retreat with my dukes up.

And Catholics also understood the psychological value of confronting death without prettying it up. At Roman Catholic wakes I had attended, a velvet kneeling bench was arranged by the open casket so visitors could touch and kiss the dead. Though agonizing, looking at death signals the beginning of grief. Thinking of "It" as a glorified tonsillectomy that had ended my "eggnancy," which was made of "a ball of cells" had been a generous gift from my psyche, but I was ready to take off the psychological training wheels. Denying the magnitude of my abortion meant denying the magnitude of my healing.

"They run one thousand of these retreats in fifty-seven countries every year," I told Greg. "In forty-eight states [Arkansas and Utah got the shaft]. They'd be shut down if spiritual abuse were an issue." I'd even searched for message board complaints online, finding nothing. Literally. Nothing but official websites.

A few days earlier, I'd bumped into a card-carrying Catholic from my Twelve Step meeting and randomly blurted out my plans to go to Rachel's Vineyard. She told me she'd signed up for the retreat a couple of years earlier but had ditched at the last minute. I couldn't believe she, of all people, had "qualified" to attend. She looked like a Republican presidential candidate—polished red suit, great dental work. *You know how there are some things you can never make right?* she'd asked. I'd nodded, but I didn't want to think having an abortion was one of those things.

Despite his father's worries, Greg seemed convinced that I would be okay, which convinced me I'd be okay, too.

I read up on the history of the retreat. In 1994, a Roman Catholic psychologist named Theresa Burke invited a group of women to a weekend of healing after abortion. She believed that a peer, a priest, and a psychologist were the holy trinity of recovery. In a YouTube video, Burke explained, "I saw very quickly that all my training in psych really didn't touch this wound. It was so deep. It was so big. It had a lot of spiritual as well as psychological components; a lot of grief, and a lot of guilt. So I saw that it needed a process of reconciliation and then I turned to the gifts in the faith to integrate them into a treatment model." I searched for a personal qualification in Burke's story to no avail.

So she started Rachel's Vineyard. The name "Rachel" came from Jeremiah 31:15–17:

> Rachel is weeping for her children;
> she refuses to be comforted for her children,
> because they are no more.
> Thus says the Lord:
> Keep your voice from weeping,
> and your eyes from tears,
> for there is a reward for your work,
> says the Lord:
> they shall come back from the land of the enemy;
> there is hope for your future.

Burke has a good story about how she came to the word "vineyard." (It's not about wine. I'm sorry.) When Burke presented the idea for Rachel's Vineyard at psychology conferences, her colleagues were adamant that she omit the religious aspects. Burke turned to her Bible for answers, opening it randomly and running her finger down the page with her eyes closed. By chance she landed at John 15:5: "I am the vine, you are the branches. Those who abide in me and I in them bear much fruit, because apart from me you can do nothing." God was the vine and Burke was a branch. Ergo, she gave us Rachel's Vineyard. (The only other time Burke did such a thing was when she was nervous about getting married and letting go of her freedom, so she opened the Bible and her finger landed on 1 Corinthians 7:9: "better to marry than to burn." She married and had five children.)

I WAITED FOR MY RIDE TO the retreat on the curb on Long Island. Trains rumbled by behind me. A mother in a hijab holding hands with her two small children moved across the parking lot. Men in suits, women in skirts and sneakers, and me, in a black bomber jacket and black cowgirl boots, wondering what the bloody hell I'd gotten myself into.

On the train, I had made the mistake of reading some of the catechism of the Catholic Church. Talk about scary: "Since the first century the Church has affirmed the moral evil of every procured abortion. This teaching has not changed and remains unchangeable." In 1869, Pope Pius IX had ruled that "ensoulment" began at conception, when egg met sperm, though Catholic doctors and theologians had debated the definition for centuries. Abortion was considered a mortal sin. Even supporting friends and partners qualified. Without a formal confession to a priest, they would (*I* would?) be banned from heaven—and the church itself: "The church attaches the canonical penalty of excommunication to this crime against human life."

Then I discovered that Burke had transferred ownership of Rachel's Vineyard to Priests for Life, an organization that runs anti-abortion campaigns. The leaders of the retreat might feel morally obliged to strong-arm us into a confession, "for our own good."

I dipped a trembling hand into my purse and pulled out a piece of white legal paper. I sat down on my duffel bag and scribbled a list of rules in preparation for my weekend stay.

Rules for Rachel's Vineyard
1. *You are a Free Agent, or: You Can Leave if You Have To*
2. *God Thinks You're Great, and God Is Bigger Than Fear*
3. *If You Feel Sad, Find Somebody Sadder Than You Are & Comfort Her as If Your Happiness Depends on It*
4. *If It Hurts Too Badly, Be a Journalist*

I stood back up and cupped my hand over my eyes to scan the parking lot for my ride. I sat back down. I stood up and took off my jacket and then put it back on. I felt like I was in the midst of a bad trip on psychedelic mushrooms. I was also starving.

A hatchback approached. A man and a woman waved at me. I waved back. They seemed nice and normal.

"I'm Corey," said the woman, stepping out of the car and opening her arms. We embraced. She had a glossed magenta bob and a tall, lean distance runner's build. She wore a cropped white jacket. "And that's Don"—she gestured to her husband as he heaved my bag into the trunk and slammed it. He looked like a Calvin Klein model from the '90s in blue jeans and a plain T-shirt with a breast pocket.

"My name's Kassi. Thanks so much for the ride. Was it too far out of your way?"

"Hours and miles," she joked. "Nah, this was easy. Just an errand for God."

What kind of God you got? I wanted to know, but didn't ask.

Inside the car, Corey turned around in the passenger's seat and grinned at me. She had a deadpan disposition, always trying to level with you.

"Been planning your escape route?" she asked, which gave me a shock. I thought of the first rule I had jotted down and felt exposed and understood, both in the same instant.

"I've got a cab on speed dial," I said.

She laughed, and I sort of laughed. Then I took a silent oath not to dial the number, partly because these people seemed relatable, but partly because I decided that the exercises in this retreat had to be part of my healing—without contempt prior to investigation. I hadn't wanted to acknowledge what had happened with a Buddhist priest, but it had ended my nightmares. I didn't want my heart to break all the way open, but I'd have to let it. I had hired these people to put a hit out on my heart. If they didn't break it, then I'd want my money back.

Corey told me that she and Don had had an abortion as high school sweethearts. When the last of their four grown children flew out of the nest, Corey was blindsided by grief over the loss of their first child, the one who hadn't been born. She signed up for Rachel's Vineyard.

"She came home a different person," said Don, looking at me through the rearview mirror.

"How so?" I asked, wanting to know what to expect. They'd had an abortion together and then married and had four children. My ex was in and out of jail with a daughter he was unprepared to be a father to. "The one who got away" was about to be legally bound to someone else, at least by a mortgage. And I couldn't stop worrying that Greg was cheating on me, this very minute. I cradled my phone, my boyfriend surveillance system, in my hand.

"The rituals just opened me up," Corey said. Don went through the program next, and now they volunteered with Rachel's Vineyard.

We entered a long asphalt driveway that appeared to have no end. Trees were planted in equidistant procession. The car rushed toward the redbrick embrace of a structure that appeared to be an elite boarding school or a country club. It was a seminary.

A breeze cooled the back of my neck as I carried my duffel bag up the regal front stoop. The door looked like the hood of a treasure chest. I studied the nameplate: Immaculate Conception.

The door opened with a creak. A thin man with wrinkles deep-baked into his face grabbed me by the shoulders and pulled me into the foyer. He pecked my cheek.

"I'm the guy you're looking for. I'm Vince." Deacon Vince. His silver hair was slicked over to the left.

"Hi. I'm Kassi," I said. Paintings the size of billboards covered the walls. Baby Jesus clinging to Mother Mary, his little bum flashing a full moon.

I hadn't been to church since I'd been pregnant.

I took my phone out of my purse to text Greg at the next possible moment, but a hand covered mine and the cell phone was snatched away. Confused, I looked from my empty hand up to a woman in her sixties standing before me, blinking behind a pair of wire-rimmed glasses. A neat strawberry blonde coif.

"No cell phones," she commanded, with a Long Island accent like Deacon Vince's. Her schoolmarm demeanor made me think she was in charge.

"I'm just—"

"This weekend is for you," she said as she turned off the phone. I wasn't sure it had ever been turned off before.

"Okay," I said, afraid of what else she'd take from me if I crossed her. Looking over my head and not at my face, she handed the phone back to me and then turned, tottering away on strappy champagne heels. I dropped it in my purse, mentally scheming to sneak away and text Greg later to check on him.

It was time for dinner; I walked down a long hallway and locked strides with a plush woman dressed in a powder blue shirt with blue lace around the neckline. In profile, she had a Roman nose. I figured one of us should say something. We each knew one personal detail about the other—that is, why we were there in the first place—but neither of us would bring it up. Ending my pregnancy had been easy to talk about as a fact of my history, but it felt different now that I was older. I felt a sense of honor and reverence toward my pregnancy that I stopped allowing myself to show after college, once I let mine get swallowed up in talk of the political machine—and before the *mizuko kuyo* ceremony.

In the cafeteria, we broke apart to load our trays without saying a word. I hungrily eyed the buffet table. A platter of turkey hoagies. Chunks of ham mixed with black beans. A bowl of potato salad laced with bacon. Not a single vegan option.

I was so famished, I wanted to grab the whole bowl of potato salad and race up to my bedroom and eat it with my bare hands. Sometimes I just wanted to be alone with bacon.

A young chef in checkered pants was leaning against a post.

"Is there any vegan food here?" I asked him.

"We don't really do vegan food here." Deacon Vince hadn't told him? "I can make you a bowl of pasta," he said. Pasta usually wasn't vegan—eggs in the noodles—but it was close enough. My adrenaline was jacked up, and I was too ravenous to work any harder for my atonement diet.

I took a seat at a round wooden table. The woman from the hallway introduced herself as Amy and then turned back to her plate. Her spoon shook. Corey and Don joined us, laughing, taking turns poking each other on the shoulder like kids. Then came a hulking priest named Father Jamie. As a Franciscan friar, he strove to emulate Jesus and Saint Francis of Assisi. Which explained why he owned nary a possession, aside from the hooded gray robe he wore every single day, belted by a natural rope. The robe was long and looked heavy, with what appeared to be a layer of soot under the sleeves. He stood about six foot five and had a scraggly beard.

"Why'd you become a priest?" I asked Father Jamie. Being a spiritual leader seemed like an inconvenient vocation in the twenty-first century.

Father Jamie had a deep, fatigued voice and bulged his eyes as if he were telling a ghost story. He told me he used to tend bar in Nevada. When he wasn't pouring shots for the locals, he tripped acid—or that's what he seemed to imply when he winked at me and said he "accessed alternate realities, and I know you know what I mean"— and made enormous potions of soymilk from scratch. He spread his giant hands to indicate the size of the tub. In another life, he could have been my boyfriend.

Father Jamie continued. Hunkered on the seat of his motorcycle, many years ago, he'd peered out at the road ahead and clenched the handlebars and headed east, driving clear across the country, promising God that if he survived the ride, he would take a vow of celibacy. Talk about a no-win situation.

Now he was in the middle of a joke. "Those folks from Corpus Christi, Texas. They say they're from Corpus, but I told 'em, guys, that's the body of Christ."

I smiled. Corey and Don ceded an encouraging chuckle. Amy gaped at her pile of potato mush and mayonnaise, looking as frightened as I was starting to feel.

Deacon Vince pulled up a chair for himself and the woman who had turned off my cell phone—his wife, Linda. Her long cotton skirt shifted over her knees as Vince pushed her up to the table.

"You don't have that cell phone, do you?" she asked me, laughing with her mouth closed. "Jesus didn't have a cell phone."

I forced myself to laugh with her. I didn't feel I was in a position not to.

"I tell ya," Deacon Vince said. "Men today should take a hint from Joseph, who stuck by his pregnant girlfriend." He was pointing his fork in the air.

"We should all take a hint," Father Jamie said, with his mouth full. "Jesus, Joseph, and Mary were illegal immigrants."

Linda shook her head, twisting her rose-stained lips. "No," she said, overflowing with confidence, "Jesus was not an illegal immigrant."

"Yes," countered Father Jamie. "Jesus was an illegal immigrant. All three of them were. They left Bethlehem to escape King Herod. Herod had it out for li'l Jesus. How'd you think the family entered Egypt?"

Linda spooned potato salad into her mouth, compulsively shaking her head.

"How'd you meet?" I asked Linda and Vince, wanting to know their backgrounds (and wanting to change the subject).

"At a Rachel's Vineyard–related presentation about a decade ago," said Linda.

She hadn't had an abortion herself, but when she was sixteen, she told me, she had become pregnant by an older man. The year was 1963, a decade before abortion became legal nationwide. "So I know what it's like to be pregnant when you don't want to be," she said to me.

Linda's family demanded that she marry the man and have the baby. When she was in her forties, after her husband had abused her for nearly three decades, she worked up the nerve to file for divorce and start over. She received a "calling" to serve the pro-life movement and attended a conference about postabortion healing, where she first laid eyes on the man who would become her second husband.

"Vince was giving a talk at the podium and I thought he was so cute. He invited me to meet him outside the abortion mill the next morning to sidewalk counsel the ladies going in. We've been together ever since."

"Sidewalk counseling" meant trying to dissuade patients from having abortions as they entered clinics. Tactics included praying loudly on the clinic grounds, calling women names, throwing baby doll parts at them, holding up picket signs with photos of blood and gore, often either digitally altered images or not even depicting abortion, and blocking the doors. Volunteers in orange or yellow vests escorted people into the facilities, sometimes meeting them at their cars and holding boom boxes to their ears to drown out the picketers.

"When did you stop 'sidewalk counseling'?" I asked, thinking surely the Church wouldn't permit a clinic picketer to run this retreat.

"We didn't stop," said Linda.

"We're still out there," said Deacon Vince. "Father Jamie, too."

I looked over at Amy to gauge her reaction to this startling information, but she appeared to be tuning out the conversation as best she could with a resolute focus on her meal. Corey and Don didn't seem the least bit fazed.

I remembered my first Rachel's Vineyard rule—You Are a Free Agent—and wanted to go AWOL. Run home. Hide under my covers with a box of Oreos.

I would spend the next forty-eight hours with three clinic picketers in a remote seminary without transportation, very few rations, and no communication with the outside world.

"These women aren't evil," said Linda, referring to the people she "sidewalk counseled," perhaps forgetting that Amy, Corey, and I were also "these women" (Don, too).

I asked Linda why she stood outside clinics and "counseled" women going in.

She answered me in a smooth cadence, complete sentences flowing as if she were writing them in cursive. "My only business, Kassi, is to be the face of Christ and to see the face of Christ in them."

THE RITUALS BEGAN AFTER DINNER. Our hub for the weekend was a circle of tall-backed needlepoint chairs and bowed couches, the scent of carnations wafting from a white flower arrangement on a shelf.

Without booze and boys, my original comforts, I sought comfort in just about anything familiar. The taste of black coffee I was sipping. The God I prayed to. The old tree outside the window. It swaying from side to side, washed in a glorious amber light, its branches like a priestess with her arms raised in the orans position, extended upward and opening.

I squeezed in next to Amy on a couch, fisting my coffee mug in one hand, dropping my purse on the floor with the other. Amy folded her hands in her lap. I wanted to befriend her. I wanted to know what she thought of this place after dinner with the protesters.

"I like your tattoo," I said, pointing at a pair of blue slippers, the size of a quarter, needled on her wrist. She quietly thanked me.

"What's its significance?" I asked, already knowing the answer. "You don't have to say if you don't want to."

"It's for my son," she told me. That son. I had thought of getting an abortion tattoo on my biceps, but held off for my mother. She would murder me if I ever walked down the aisle with ink on my arm.

I was geared up to ask Amy more about herself when a man in a pastel tartan shirt hustled in the room, issuing an apologetic wave for being late. His entrance prompted a blonde with windswept hair to slump over in her chair. Father Jamie laid the weight of his arm around her shoulders and leaned over to offer inaudible words of consolation as she wept into her trembling hands. Her fingernails were painted bubble gum pink. The man walked over and knelt down before the woman. The two whispered loud enough for me to ascertain that they attended the same church. She was afraid the man would out her to their small clan for being seen at this retreat. They whispered back and forth and seemed to establish an agreement.

"Welcome, welcome," said the mellifluent voice of Linda. Amy and I cranked our heads to the left. Linda was running her fingernails through her peach-colored hair, a three-ring binder in her lap. The man darted to a seat. Two other men who'd been arm-wrestling on a side table with Don dispersed and then gathered in the circle.

Six leaders staffed the retreat, with four additional rotating facilitators. I was relieved that three of the leaders—Corey, her husband Don, and a newlywed in her thirties—had experienced abortion personally, though I had expected that to be a basic qualification. The other three main staff members were clinic picketers.

Nine retreat participants were present—three men and six women. Such a high ratio of leaders to participants could easily affect the dynamics of the group. At twenty-five years old, I was the youngest person in attendance. A grandmother in her sixties was the oldest.

"This is our twenty-fifth weekend retreat," Linda gushed. "We have memorialized more than five hundred aborted babies. Very exciting!!!" She burst into a country club clap and nodded her head, cuing the rest of us to applaud. I hesitantly clapped my hands.

Corey rolled out a television set. Over the next twenty minutes, a grainy VHS disseminated misleading medical information about abortion. The narrator, a woman wearing shoulder pads that extended from coast to coast, claimed that abortion heightened the risk of breast cancer (the best studies disagree, but most conclude that breast cancer and abortion are not related), postabortion syndrome (make believe), and infertility (rare, but not impossible). When the movie ended, I hoped Corey would give a disclaimer explaining that the information was in direct conflict with the medical community, but she didn't. Nobody did.

Amy raised her hand and told the group that she had the "syndrome." *Oh, no,* I thought. *I'm losing Amy.* Then a tall redhead shared that she had survived breast cancer years ago and now she knew what caused it. *Oh, no,* I thought. *I'm losing everybody.* I couldn't take at face value a video with a clear political and religious bias, with no basis in sound scientific methodology.

But even "scientific studies" validated by the secular establishment could be biased, funded by special-interest groups, and full of nonsense.

Amy and I talked in the hall after Linda released us for a short break. "I know the syndrome's not real," she told me, not whispering, but not speaking at a normal volume, either. I was relieved. "It's just that nobody else would believe me when I told them I thought about my son all the time. I'd be sitting at my work computer, knowing my co-workers would think I was a lunatic if I told them."

The muscle in my chest gripped. Noah's Jade was almost three.

Father Jamie beckoned to us. "I want to show you something," he said, and Amy and I followed him down a long hallway, flanked by portraits of priests, and out the front doors of the seminary.

I shivered in the night air, rubbing my arms as we trudged onto the lawn. The trees rustled in the wind. Father Jamie stuck his hand in the marsupial pouch of his robe, the sleeves fluttering, and dug around until he pulled out a tiny plastic fetus. I turned away.

"Consider this your formal invitation to confession," he said with a bearded grin. "You can tell me anything. You can even confess that you murdered someone. Then, I'll say"—he laid one gargantuan hand on Amy's head—"YOU HAVE BEEN ABSOLVED."

Amy, strands of her beach-colored hair hanging over her face, nodded to indicate that the invitation had been received. Father Jamie moseyed across the lawn but the two of us hung back.

"Are you okay?" I asked.

"Yeah," she said. "That was pretty dumb."

"So you gonna make confession?" I asked, half-joking.

"Yeah," she said. I was stunned, my mouth agape. "There's nowhere else to go," she continued. "It wouldn't be a popular opinion here, but I'm pro-choice. I just made the wrong choice."

"I feel naïve admitting to this," I said, conspiratorially, "but I thought they used 'murder' for lack of a better word. This is such an awkward dynamic."

"I'll do anything it takes to feel better. If it's confession, I'll go."

I'd do almost anything, too, but I wouldn't sit in a confessional with a man who carried a plastic fetus in his pocket to try to guilt me into telling him my secret thoughts about my dead baby.

"Thank God you're here," I said. Amy made me want to stay. She and I walked through the dark back toward the seminary, its windows black, the lights out everywhere but that little room.

WE EACH HAD TWENTY MINUTES to tell our stories—*exactly* twenty minutes, decreed by the plastic kitchen timer in Deacon Vince's hand.

Amy went first. Her eyes were puffy, her curls arranged carefully over her shoulders.

"I got pregnant sixteen years ago, and everything just got turned around." She had a Long Island accent with an *I've had it* baseline. "I just don't remember how. I never saw Dave again—that's the guy's name. We had been together for three years. I was calling him, calling him . . . he never answered me. Then, it was like I got up off the couch and never spoke of it again. You pretend it never happened so you don't have to deal with it. You don't even know you're doing it. Six months later, I met my husband and got pregnant with my daughter." She laced her fingers, long painted nails, looked down at them thoughtfully.

"I joined Facebook and friended Dave and remembered that he was supposed to be the love of my life. He saw a photo of my daughter, and he asked if she was his." Her face blanched. "Sometimes I want to drive into the middle of traffic. I told my therapist it was my main issue, but she doesn't get it. She understands emotions like loss and regret but has never understood how abortion could cause those things."

"Wait a minute, she didn't understand how an abortion could cause those things?"

This came from Dr. Lou, mid-fifties, a Roman Catholic psychologist in a tweed jacket whose role was to interpret our testimonies, with his pitchy, exasperated tenor that reminded me of Ned Flanders of *The Simpsons,* which was endearing. Dr. Lou said he and his wife had had eighteen (eighteen!) children, but only eight of them had survived in the womb and been born.

Amy licked her lips and shook her head no.

Dr. Lou pretended to pull out his feathered hair. "Therapists aren't properly trained to recognize the symptoms of postabortion syndrome. I tried to offer a training to psychology interns, but my idea was shot down."

Deacon Vince, sitting to the left of us with his legs spread out like a cowboy's, declared "TIME." He crossed his arms over his head like a referee.

I patted Amy's shoulder as she dabbed her cheeks with a tissue, turning toward the couch to hide her face and then back to the circle. "I want Dave to know that I love and miss our son," she said. "I will never forget our son."

Vince reset the kitchen timer.

"Okay," said Linda. "Steve?"

I had five years sober; Steve had twenty. He was tall and sixty years old with a handsome symmetrical face, slate gray hair and a news anchor inflection. Steve began nodding, as if the story was buried deep down inside him and he had to crank it up to the surface like well water. I couldn't help but think I was hearing Noah's side of the story. I wondered how he felt when the pregnancy entered his mind, if it entered his mind at all, how maybe he shoved it down with a syringe.

"I had as much influence as she did in the decision to terminate, so there's no energy going on about me blaming her or her blaming me. It's not one of those things," he said, his whole mouth quivering. "We got married a few years later, but when we wanted kids, she had ectopic pregnancies. So the only child we ever could have had was the one we aborted. We came close to an adoption, but we had anxiety. There was a big scare on fetal alcohol poisoning in Russia, where we were looking. I think I just wanted my baby back. The worst thing about it was my indifference when it was going on. I was twenty-seven. I was just like, yeah, you do that, you go to the clinic, and then we'll get a cheeseburger. When I was able to look at it, having gotten sober and everything, I could see—" His voice cracked. "Man, how can a person be like that?"

He tried to continue his story. He lifted a finger, begging a moment to regain his composure, but a minute later, his chin fell to his chest and he wept.

Noah hadn't been a rock of support, but he hadn't been indifferent, either. I remember lying on his mattress, nauseated and exhausted, while his phone blew up with calls from his buddies, offering help and money. I couldn't get him to stop telling people I was pregnant. His prepster redheaded drug dealer roommate came in eating a cold slice of pizza. From the vantage of the bed, I watched him laugh a cocky laugh, saying what a cute kid it'd be, and a mistake. Noah wouldn't take help or money, and he wouldn't stop telling everyone. The thing about Noah's Facebook photos was that he looked like a "good father" when he wasn't locked up. It was obvious that Jade adored him, lived for him, in every photo was pointing at him or squeezing him the way a kid hugs a Disney World cartoon character they might never meet again. Jade and Noah mugged the camera in matching gray ski hats. In a plain white T-shirt with stenciled sleeve tattoos, Noah carried Jade on his shoulders, and she clasped his forehead with both hands.

Linda authorized a break, and the circle slowly scattered. I struck up a conversation with Steve by the snack table, asking him whether he believed his wife's termination had caused his alcoholism. It was an idea that contradicted the dominant recovery belief that no one and nothing was to blame for our addiction. Steve shook his head and said he didn't buy in to the syndrome, but he thought the abortion had "pushed" his alcoholism, had accelerated his drinking. I could say the same—having an abortion helped me hit bottom and get sober much faster.

Had mine pushed a syringe of heroin into Noah's arm?

I powerwalked down the hall with my phone and hid in the windowless bathroom to sneak a Google of Noah's police log. As if our lives were in cosmic conversation, he had been arrested that day, charged with possession of cocaine. I had walked into a seminary; he had walked into a jail cell. I was about to text Greg, but there was a knock on the door.

"You okay, Kassi?" It was Corey.

"I'm good," I said, slipping my phone in my pocket, not sure how long I'd been in there.

TESSA AND ABE WERE THE ONLY COUPLE attending Rachel's Vineyard together as participants. Abe wore baggy black pants and a standard issue green T-shirt, size XXL on his size S frame. He had a small face with a small nose, and eyes like bullet heads. Dressed in a black hoodie, black skinny jeans, and black sneakers, Tessa was shaped like a chalice. A shadowy bun was stacked on top of her head. Big bright eyes, plump lips.

Their social worker had sent them to the retreat. Tessa's story wasn't the typical tale from the clinic, although she said she'd had four or five abortions in the past. She was here because she'd miscarried at six months and was potentially facing murder charges.

"I was having migraines, high blood pressure, swollen feet and legs," said Tessa. "It was hard to work, so I lost my job. I didn't want to tell my boss about the pregnancy, especially if it was going to be adopted."

Tessa said the baby looked like an eggplant. "I had my sister drive me to the hospital because I didn't want to draw attention to my apartment," she said. "The cops showed up in my hospital room. They accused me of murder. I told them the baby came out on its own. I'd left the baby at home. It could change everything. I could lose everything."

"I was almost home," Abe cut in.

Tessa slapped his bare arm with a quick reflex.

"Abe's time frame is always off. He went home and got the baby and brought the baby to the hospital. He was telling the cops he came home an hour later, which made it seem like he waited at home for a while before he came to the hospital. I couldn't get dressed, and so I just got in the bath. I called someone who knew me—my sister. The cops thought I did the wrong thing."

A priest swayed back and forth in a rocking chair, angling his face in such a way that the interior of his nose was visible. He was dressed in a clerical collar, his jet-black hair slicked with Brylcreem. Linda introduced him as a twenty-year veteran of pro-life activism.

"You'd rather jeopardize the life of the baby than call an ambulance," he said.

"The baby wasn't alive," she reminded him.

"The hospital could have saved him if you'd called the ambulance," he said.

Tessa ignored him. "The cops put crime scene tape over the front door and searched my apartment while I was in the hospital. I got the ashes. We had a ceremony."

"TIME," hollered Deacon Vince. He stood up with his wrists crossed over his head again.

"I'm here to forgive myself," Tessa said.

A tissue box made its way around the circle.

Linda turned to me. I crossed my legs and sat up straight.

The rotten priest had left, thank goodness, but I was still hesitant to talk. I'd seen how it worked. We told our stories, and then the leaders said: "The question is, what led you to make this unhealthy choice?" I was afraid of what they'd say to me, because I was afraid of what I would say back.

I didn't use the word "baby" or even "water baby." I tried not to cry because I didn't want my tears to be mistaken as a justification for picketing or "sidewalk counseling."

I bullet-pointed my story, told them my mom invited me to move home and have the baby. "The grandmotherly instinct kicked in!" said Dr. Lou. That was one way of looking at it.

I told them that my boss at the vintage store, Dez, had pointed out that my life was no place for a child, and that it would have been selfish of me to continue the pregnancy just to avoid feeling guilty about ending it. Linda, Dr. Lou, Vince, and Father Jamie shook their heads no in unison.

Either way I chose, I was selfish according to somebody. If I had a baby at twenty years old, shame on me for messing up my life. If I had an abortion, shame on me for messing up someone else's life. If I adopted out, shame on me for depleting the resources for millions of orphans and billions of people on the overpopulated planet. There is no choice a woman can make without somebody thinking she should be doing something else. It was becoming clear to me that the one voice I could trust is the voice of my most faithful, fearless, self.

"The last time I saw Noah, two years ago, he'd overdosed on heroin in a Starbucks bathroom," I managed. "Now he's in jail."

A few people gasped. Dr. Lou's jaw flopped open. Linda straightened her glasses. Somebody passed me the box of tissues.

"Noah has a child now."

I'd always wondered how Jade's mother had persuaded Noah to support her having the baby, wished I could've eavesdropped on the conversation. I wanted to know what he said when his (ex) girlfriend told him the test was positive. That he wasn't ready? Did she say, *Too bad*? Had our abortion changed him? Did she know about it? Were they trying to have a baby?

"She's almost three years old," I continued. "His daughter wouldn't exist if I'd had a baby with him."

Abe and Tessa gave me a solidarity nod. Linda sat perfectly still, wire-rimmed glasses pinching her nose.

"Our objective, Kassi," Linda said, "is to help you realize that a child has died."

I wanted to say, *I know, Linda. It was mine. I was there. I had it sucked out of me for four hundred and fifteen bucks. I think of it every hour. I drank over it, blew cocaine over it, bought a key chain of a bust with an embryo, hung up a print of a Wonder Woman with an umbilical cord instead of a Lasso of Truth. But there's a difference between a dead child and an unlived life.*

I wanted to say, *My objective, Linda, is to help you realize a child has also lived.*

"You are a mother and will be until the day you die." Linda spoke slowly so I could swallow every word. "You can't deny it. You can't say it's not a part of who you are."

I thought I'd blast out of my body when she told me that. The kitchen timer beeped.

"THE TIME HAS COME FOR THE STONING RITUAL," Linda said, holding up a gray stone the size of a potato.

A stoning ritual sure sounded dangerous, but I liked the Bible story this ritual was based on. An adulteress is forced to stand up straight in front of Jesus. The teachers of the law try to get Jesus to agree with them that she should be stoned for disgracing her husband. Jesus draws a line in the sand with his finger. Then he says, "Let anyone among you who is without sin be the first to throw a stone at her." The people walk away and he says, "Has no one condemned you?"

"No one, sir," the woman says.

"Neither do I condemn you," Jesus says. "Go your way, and from now on, do not sin again."

Linda passed the stone to Deacon Vince to demonstrate the ritual: she asked him if anyone was here to condemn him. He said no, and she told him not to sin again. Waiting for the stone to circle around to me, I kept thinking, *yeah, Linda, seems there are people here to condemn us.*

Linda gestured toward a wooden coffee table, piled with rocks like hers. "If you are carrying feelings of condemnation and think you can't be forgiven, go ahead and pick up a rock."

Jesus had drawn a line in the sand to keep the teachers of the law from judging the adulteress, but in an ironic role reversal, U.S. lawmakers had established buffer zones around abortion clinic entrances, legal "lines in the sand," to keep Christian "sidewalk counselors" from taunting people the same way I imagined the townspeople taunting the adulteress.

"Keep this rock with you all weekend," Linda continued. "Everyone will hold you accountable for bringing your rock with you. Drop the rock when you feel forgiven."

I thought, *Why don't you carry your own Rock of Shame and why don't you drop the rock when you're done condemning us?*

I selected a rock with a pale purple sheen. It was cold and heavy, seven pounds or so, the weight of a newborn.

I eased back into my seat next to Amy, reaching down to stuff the purple Rock of Shame in my handbag. Before I could sit up straight, I was nearly launched off the couch. Linda had sat down hard between Amy and me with a buttery smile. Her lips were painted coral pink. She was holding a bottle of wine in one hand and a glass pitcher in the other.

"Next up is the Cup of Bitterness," she announced, holding up the bottle. Four of us in attendance were ex-drunks—she assured us that the bottle was filled with grape juice and not wine. She handed me the bottle and then held out the pitcher in front of me.

"Kassi, share with us what you're angry at. Say, 'Into this pitcher, I pour out my bitterness at the evils of Planned Parenthood abortion mills and the lies liberal politicians tell.' Or whomever you're mad at. Then pass it on."

I balanced the bottle on one of my legs. Linda was close enough to touch me, close enough that I could feel her body heat. I didn't want to be enraged, but I was totally enraged. I knew enough not to pull a Jesus and flip tables, but I didn't have the power to make my anger disappear. I felt like a dink for expecting these people to be of the Catholics for Choice variety. I decided to participate just enough to complete the exercise and get upstairs to reunite with my own God in private—the one from Rule 2 who Thinks I'm Great and Is Bigger Than Fear.

"So I just say what I'm angry about?" I asked, stalling.

Don nodded at me. "Talk about your anxieties and stuff like that," he said.

I was so frazzled that I tipped the bottle and blurted out, "Into this pitcher, I pour my bitterness . . . toward anxiety."

Don't ask me what that meant because I've got no idea.

The bottle hopped to the next lap.

With the pressure off, I could think about bitterness. I doodled in a small spiral notebook in my lap until a crude pencil drawing emerged of a face—my face—with zits. After Noah had emailed me about Jade, cystic acne turned my chin and right cheek into a topographic map, all the zits blending together into lumpy patches of skin. Needless to say, I felt gorgeous. I'd hardly had a pimple in high school and college. None of my high school beauty research prepared me to cure my acne. Just when I had guzzled carrot juice by the liter (and then worried about my skin turning orange), eliminated dairy from my diet (going completely vegan), washed my face with cucumber juice, drunk gallons of water, slept nine hours a night, and swallowed an antibiotic that gave me flulike aches and chills, a Buddhist lama on a podcast explained that the spiritual cause of acne was pent-up rage.

By then, the acne had cleared up because I was suffering through the antibiotics side effects, but I never forgot about the suggestion that fury had ruined my face.

I pretended I didn't have any resentment at Noah, because I was so spiritual, you see. But there was a delicate balance between spiritual maturity and emotional responsibility. Spiritual maturity means choosing not to blame other people for my problems. Emotional responsibility means bucking up and addressing my feelings and behavior when other people have an effect on me.

Deacon Vince shuffled around with a steeple of Dixie cups, and Don followed with bitterness on tap.

"To bitterness," thundered Father Jamie. We lifted our cups.

MY BEDROOM WAS ALL BED AND BREAKFAST, all chestnut wood and pastel quilts. A white geranium bloomed in a terracotta pot. Gifts were spread around the room—a lavender bag set on an antique writing table, a small knit blanket on the bed, a stack of typewritten notes from various members of the clergy. I shuffled through the notes and stopped when I came to a letter from Pope John Paul II:

> *The Church is aware of the many factors which may have influenced your decision, and she does not doubt that in many cases it was a painful and even shattering decision. The wound in your heart may not yet have healed. Certainly what happened was and remains terribly wrong. But do not give in to discouragement and do not lose hope. Try rather to understand what happened and face it honestly. If you have not already done so, give yourselves over with humility and trust to repentance. The Father of mercies is ready to give you his forgiveness and his peace in the Sacrament of Reconciliation. To the same Father and His mercy you can with sure hope entrust your child.*
>
> EVANGELIUM VITAE. 25 MARCH 1995.

The window overlooked a dark spread of land, half a mile from the ocean, and let in an earthy breeze.

The lavender gift bag contained Mary Kay cosmetics, which I pulled out one by one: a pot of face cream, a tube of lip gloss, a container of blush, a pallet of eye shadow, a bronzer. Then a stretchy black shirt that was an odd hybrid of exercise gear and business casual. White print on the neckline read: "Uniting to be Smoke-Free," all part of a broad-sweeping effort to extend life.

Sitting on the twin bed, I shook out the blanket. It was Coke brown and Slurpee blue. A note from the knitter explained that she had been praying for me while she worked on this "shawl." I couldn't help noticing that it could double as a newborn's blanket—or my new Forgiveness Cape. I wrapped it around my shoulders. Anger radiated off of me like steam.

I imagined marching out of this room and bursting into the chapel and reporting in a loud voice that I did not intend to worship a pregnant teen virgin or to confess murder to a priest who carried a plastic fetus in his pocket. Going to the chapel to tell Corey how uncomfortable I felt seemed like precisely the thing to do to rid myself of anger. I pulled on my boots and stomped down the narrow hall to tell Corey I had lied. I had bitterness, and it wasn't just toward "anxiety." I trusted Corey: she had had an abortion.

I swung open the heavy chapel door, which fanned the darkness with light. The scent of spiced incense hung in the air. A hundred feet away, Corey was a shadow on her knees, running a long string of rosary beads through her hands. Afraid I'd caught her in a private moment, I waited in a pew by the door, hoping I could confess my thoughts to her, hoping she could convey a spiritual logic that would make sense to me.

Candles flickered on the altar. Behind it, a fuzzy line of figures in the choir's pews. Ten minutes passed before Corey stood. A staunch bow to the crucifix, then she turned on her heel. When she walked by me, I opened my mouth but nothing came out. Not a word. Corey didn't look over at me. The door closed. I wanted to follow her, but I was still frozen on the pew, unable to speak.

I returned to my room and sat on the bed with my notebook in my lap. A line is drawn in the sand. "Let anyone among you who is without sin be the first to throw a stone at her."

I placed my stone on the bed and picked up my pen and wrote my anger.

They are so dogmatic and judgmental. They think they're more spiritually advanced than I am. They are more interested in reinforcing their own deep-seated judgments than in helping us heal. They don't want to listen to us. They want to control us and tell our stories for us.

Then, I crossed out "They" and wrote "I."

~~They are~~ I am so dogmatic and judgmental. ~~They think they're~~ I think I'm more spiritually advanced than ~~I am~~ they are. ~~They are~~ I am more interested in reinforcing ~~their own~~ my own deep-seated judgments than in helping ~~us~~ myself heal. ~~They don't~~ I don't want to listen to ~~them~~ us. ~~They want~~ I want to control ~~us~~ them and tell their story for them ~~our stories for us~~.

Buddha was disguised as a Roman Catholic.
I continued:

Any word I say, any gesture, any emotion in my voice could be distorted and read as evidence of my guilt. The guilt they ascribe to me. It feels like a prison for my words and actions to be under the microscope.

Then I crossed out "I" and wrote "Greg."

Any word I Greg says, any gesture, any emotion in my his voice could be distorted and read as evidence of my his guilt. The guilt they I ascribe to me him. It feels like a prison for my his words and actions to be under the microscope.

Poor Greg.

It was 3 A.M. I kneeled and set my elbows on the bed and clasped my hands.

It's me, God. It's all me. Well, not all me, but a sizable portion. May I forgive myself for being so dogmatic, judgmental, and suspicious. Please help me to listen, tell the truth, and trust—and even if I can't trust them, help me to trust myself to handle tough stuff. May Linda and everyone I see as my "protesters," in whatever form they take, be happy. May Greg be free. Please show me what I can do for them both.

Amen.

Three hours later, I popped out of bed like I was coming up from under water—I was late for morning Mass. I ran into the shower, undressing midstride. Then, twisting my wet hair up in a towel, I stepped into a pair of white pants, jumping up and down.

Then I dropped my Rock of Shame to the floor.

SECRET INVISIBLE BABY FRIEND

SIX YEARS, ONE MONTH, TWO WEEKS, AND ONE DAY AFTER-
WARD—I lowered myself into a needlepoint chair. Organ music
played softly from a boom box on a shelf. The retreat participants
and leaders filed into the room, with Linda and Deacon Vince taking up the rear, each of them finding a seat in the circle. There was
buzz around the next ritual—the Living Water ritual. It was Saturday
night, the last night of what felt like a very long, very strange trip. I
had crossed the threshold only yesterday.

Linda, in a chair directly across the room from me, tapped her
tattered Bible with a pen. "We will now meet our children by naming
them," she announced.

Trying to pretend I hadn't heard that, I picked at my thumbnail,
but a noble voice without a sound told me to stay, listen, and name
the unlived life. I didn't want to, but I had to. I had to own my power
of life and of death like a savage, a brute, a woman. *Somebody who
should have been born is gone,* wrote the poet Anne Sexton in "The Abortion" in 1962.

Linda continued: "It is difficult to grieve someone we have never
met, a child with no name, and begin to mourn, like we would mourn
anyone we have lost."

She instructed us to walk to the center of the circle one by one, light a floating candle for each water baby, and release it into a bowl of "living water."

Steve hovered over the table in a checkered button-down, his back to me. He picked a votive candle from a tray. Deacon Vince fired up the lighter—*schk-schk-schk*. Reciting Linda's script, Steve said, "Lord Jesus, I pour out my heart to you, and I give you Corrine."

Cupping the candle in his hands, he released it into the water and watched his water baby float.

Everyone else named their children at the water. Nobody else showed much emotion. I had been the stoic one while everyone else wept. But now each beat of my heart seemed to deliver an electric shock of burning pain, shooting from heart to fingertips.

I can't do this ritual, I thought.

The room strobed with all the names on fire. Linda, her face flashing, called on me. I autopiloted my way center circle. At the bowl of water, I picked up a tea candle and held it in front of me, watching the orange flame climb the wick.

"God," I said, but the next words could not leave my mouth or the bomb would go off.

Linda thought I had forgotten the script: "It goes, Lord. Jesus. I—"

"God"—I interrupted her—"I pour out my heart to you, and I give you . . . Judah." A variation on the name Jade.

I set the candle in the water. And then I fell apart, sobbing uncontrollably. I choked and wailed, actually wailed. The bomb was a gush of tears and snot.

Father Jamie was sitting next to me and pinched a wad of tissues over my chair. I grabbed them from him and collapsed in the seat, crying for Judah.

You know, the fourth son of Jacob by Leah.

Linda blinked at me from behind her wire glasses.

"Kassi, how did you feel about the ritual?"

Her lips were slightly parted. I gasped for air, but it felt like there was a fist in my throat.

I jockeyed a few syllables: "A toughie," I said.

"What?" She cupped one ear.

"A TOUGHIE," said Amy, Tessa, Abe, Steve, and the others—and I loved them all.

Father Jamie stood up and gave Amy his seat. She silently held a box of Kleenex for me in her lap.

It wasn't naming the baby that felt so unbearable. What made my brain split apart was the thought of "giving the baby back to God."

It registered to me as if they were saying: give your very motivation for living back to God.

Because guilt seemed to imply wrongdoing, my ego had constructed a strong wall of defense. My guilt masqueraded as ambition and achievement and two 401Ks and promotions at work and an Ivy League admissions letter. With a shadow of guilt in my passenger's seat, I sped toward an unreachable horizon. Slow down, and I wasted two lives.

That's the price I paid: a debt as big as a life. I had to live big enough for two.

Enter the Living Water ritual. It felt like God was tapping me on the shoulder, saying, *I hate to break it to you, Kass, but the debt doesn't exist. You owe nothing. Maybe I can convince you if we act this out. Pretend that candle's a baby. Put the candle in the "Living Water." Let go.*

Why would I let go? Debt got me to Italy. Debt got me sober. Debt got me into Columbia. (In more ways than one.) Debt had never given me a Sabbath or a tropical vacation or a lazy afternoon on a front porch swing in the middle of nowhere, but without debt, what was the point in anything? Debt had been getting me out of bed in the morning since I was nineteen years old. It was the most relentless motivation I had ever known.

————————

I LINED UP BEHIND THE GROUP, holding a five-inch terrycloth doll to represent the baby. We were all holding terrycloth dolls, which came in various representations of skin pigmentation. Honoring the reverent silence—by which I mean I was just unable to speak—I followed Father Jamie and Deacon Vince as they marched us through corridors, carrying the bowl of water babies above their heads like a torch.

We descended into the stairwell and flushed out into an underground sanctuary. I followed the mourners through a black wrought-iron gate and into a small chapel filled with people I had never seen before. They were family members my cohort had invited to the service. They greeted their kin with long, silent embraces while I slid gingerly into a seat and looked at the walls: frescoes of Jesus alongside pink-winged angels.

A sash of smoke wafted from the altar and wove around a tall vase of white roses. It spread out in a fog at the front of the room. We formed a line and ceremoniously laid our dolls to rest in two wooden cribs. I pulled down a kneeling bench to pray before a crib, just like one might kneel before a casket at a wake.

As I stood up, a volcanic wail gathered in my throat. But before anyone could catch me crying and misinterpret my tears, I covered my face with my hands and made a beeline for the bathroom.

I bent over the sink, splashing my face with cold water, trying to wash off the grief. I spun away from the mirror, clutching a damp brown paper towel, embarrassed to observe my own self crying over a damn baby doll. That was not my baby, I told myself. It was a doll. I told myself that this weeping jag was completely out of proportion with an embryo the size of a lima bean.

Not helping.

I must be crying because of this, and this, and this, and maybe it's the room temperature, or I'm probably just hungry. I wished my brain would hush. Because fingers and toes weren't nothing, and for once, here, the consensus was, it wasn't nothing.

So many clashing emotions: grief over the loss of a son or daughter assembling itself. Guilt in the form of striving. Fierce resistance to the belief that abortion was wrong. Was it wrong? Table that. Return to right and wrong later.

For now, six years of sludge had to blast up and out of my body. I had an urge to hold a terribly tiny thing in the palm of my hand, and tell it, *Please, please forgive me.*

Part of me felt compassion for myself, like *Listen, girlfriend. God held out his hand and offered you a gift. A baby. He thought you wanted it! You thought about motherhood enough when you were a teenager. You thought the gift was a bit too big to fit in your life at the time. It was like somebody giving you a pony in college: you have no money, no time, and no place to keep it. Only it was an unfathomably bigger deal than a pony. You said no. God had no opinion on this. God just held out another hand and gave you another gift. God has infinite hands and opens them up compulsively, right now, all the time. God ain't checking the mail for a thank-you note or a letter of apology. God just wants you to be happy and free.*

This is where I admitted that the opposite of freedom is the one thing I didn't want to give up. It was debt.

I CLUTCHED THE LAVENDER GIFT BAG in my lap, sitting in Dr. Lou's minivan. The retreat was over. I was trembling with hunger and on the brink of tears. Dr. Lou parked the van alongside the railroad tracks. A warm wave of relief washed over me when my boots hit the pavement.

"Hey, come on down to the clinic," Dr. Lou said through the passenger's side window as I stood with my duffel over one shoulder, clutching my lavender bag by its neck. The bag contained a rolled-up set of affidavits to sign and send to Congress stating that abortion had hurt us—and that it should be illegal. "We hold vigil and do sidewalk counseling. We could sure use you there. And don't forget to sign those affidavits."

"Hmmm . . . ," I said, feeling almost swollen with pain. "Thanks for the ride."

I turned around and raced up the steps of the train platform, delirious with hunger.

- 10 -

THIRTY SECONDS OF GRIEF

SIX YEARS AND TWO MONTHS AFTERWARD—An altar was taking shape in my office. You'd think I'd found religion, what with the navy blue meditation cushion, flag for Guiding Light, and Living Water, which came in a translucent bottle emblazoned with a metallic gold cross. Maybe I needed to commit a petty theft to restore the balance. But the rituals themselves felt like lovely little rebellions against the part of me that wanted to settle for half-hearted happiness.

Remembering Guiding Light gave me peace of mind. The Living Water reminded me to let go of the idea of a "debt" and start my day with a full tank of enoughness—owing nothing, needing nothing, being satisfied. Easier said than done. The tank was usually rattling empty by lunch, but I tried my best not to try to fill the tank with unleaded attention from the male species (a key contributing factor to my pregnancy and my favorite intoxicant second to whiskey).

Miraculously, I hadn't accused Greg of a single affair since my slapdash forgiveness exercise in my bedroom at the seminary. It had been two weeks. I had resolutely turned to the "Living Water." Which is to say that I resolutely sat on the navy blue meditation cushion and asked God the subtextual questions I had been asking Greg: "Will you please be my God? Will you make me feel safe? Will you make me feel like I am enough?" (Stay tuned for my new article, "3 Flirty

Questions To Ask A Guy.") I wanted to feel so enough that anyone within a hundred mile radius of me would feel like they were enough, too. I wanted to bring this enoughness to California with me—my plane would leave in a few hours—but I had just discovered a hitch in the practice.

The Living Water had over-delivered. Now I had more than enough. I had *too much.*

It began with a nightmare about Will-B: It wasn't a subtle one, either. I'd crashed his wedding to Sarah. I barged into the chapel hideously underdressed, wearing a pair of cutoff jean shorts and no shoes, and shouted: *Wait! Don't! I'm ready now!*

In the morning—when the dream was over—I sat at my desk to take care of some last-minute correspondence before my flight, and there, at the top of my message box, was an email from Will-B. As if my nightmare had conjured him. I braced myself for news that he was married—"Yay!" I'd write back, oh, f*cking yay—but he hadn't gotten hitched. Instead, he and Sarah had parted ways. He wrote: "I often find that you are in my thoughts which is kind've [sic] weird because we haven't really seen each other much of [sic] the past decade." (Except, of course, for our yearlong romance.)

I almost turned into soft serve. Perhaps reading too much into a throwaway line dashed off in a casual email (or not?), I wondered what Will-B meant and why he would write me now, of all times, when I was in the midst of a "journey." But thoughts of him played on a loop in my head, and now, at long last, I had a rare opening to tell him so.

I assumed the position: back straight, legs crossed, hands on keyboard, primed to write back: *ditto.* Greg knew of my preoccupation with Will-B. I had made a big nervous confession at some point earlier in the year, standing in front of him, wringing my hands. Greg, seated at the kitchen table in a flannel shirt, a cigarette behind his

ear, lifted his head from the valley of a paperback and said something along the lines of, "Will-*B*? Hm. Interesting name," and then
returned to the book.

Now, looking up from my computer screen, I reached for the warm
mug of coffee Greg was delivering to me with his familiar hands.
Who was better than Greg? He was my home, I told myself. This was
my writing desk, my room with a view of the airshaft. That was my
navy blue meditation cushion.

That enormous black suitcase by the door was my bag packed for
California.

I followed Greg, who was wheeling my giant luggage, outside to
hail a cab. On the curb, I gripped his shirt with both hands and
kissed him before I sat down in the backseat of my taxi.

MY MOTHER SHOWED UP IN THE San Diego airport with her hair
landscaped to blonde perfection. We hugged, swaying side to side,
while she whispered into my ear, "Why is there a dark streak in your
hair?" It was a rhetorical question. The streak had been there for two
years.

In the rental parking garage we climbed into a pearl white Jeep
that looked like it had come rolling off the set of an adventure chick
flick. My mother wanted to persuade me that we were on a carefree
mother-daughter road trip; I hoped I wouldn't break down in front
of her—she was a bit of a drill sergeant when I cried in front of her.
"Cut the sissy shit. You'll never get anywhere in life if you can't pull
yourself together."

The shadow of the parking garage rolled over the windshield and
then sunlight flashed in our eyes. Palm fronds hung over the road
and made the sunlight a constant flicker against my sunglasses while
I shuttled us through San Diego.

We drove to the Hotel del Coronado, known as the Del, a beautiful old seaside resort with pointed red Victorian rooftops. In the lobby, a chandelier the size of a motorboat hung over my head. The woven rug under my boots could have covered the entire square footage of my Manhattan apartment. I felt I didn't deserve my mother spoiling me with an extravagant oceanfront hotel. People would be disgusted that healing after my abortion involved complimentary fruit plates and flutes of sparkling water. Then I thought, is your God "Disgusted People," or is your God a "Compulsive Giver of Gifts"? Do you really think God wants recovery to be all Anne Sexton poetry and crib memorials? Not my God.

Palm trees towered overhead and the hotel wait staff lingered nearby in black uniforms. Mom and I lounged on two lawn chairs, shivering by the pool in the cold sun. We were disappointed that California was so cold at the end of June. We had been misinformed about the weather. We had packed bathing suits. We wore matching bathrobes, too, and our heads were swathed in towels smelling of eucalyptus. Sipping a mug of hot tea with mint, I gazed at my mother through a giant pair of sunglasses while she dodged all talk of my abortion and updated me on Rusty's wedding plans—at age twenty-three, tracking our parents' marital age, he had proposed at Christmas to a girl from Detroit who was unanimously considered "a class act."

Then, overhearing the waiters talk about two well-documented suicides of pregnant women at the Del in the late 1800s, I excused myself and padded over in flip-flops to quiz them. They told me that the first woman checked into the hotel under an alias after she divulged to her lover that she was pregnant with their child. The man didn't want her to have the baby, so she supposedly attempted an abortion by drinking a bottle of quinine. In the version of the story the waiters relayed, Kate Morgan then walked out on the beach and shot herself. In another version of the story, records indicated that the bullet in her head didn't match the bullets in her gun, which would mean that someone else's gun must have discharged the fatal bullet. That version holds that she bought a gun intending to shoot her lover on the beach, but instead he pulled out his own gun and killed her first. The second woman, nameless, allegedly having an affair, reportedly killed herself in Room 3502 because she didn't want to be pregnant.

Walking back to our hotel room with towels wrapped around our waists, my mother and I passed a cake-topper bride and groom posing inside a white gazebo, both smiling sleepily for a photographer crouched at their feet.

"Kass, Kass, look," said my mother, gesturing to the polished couple.

"I see them," I replied, keeping my pace.

"How do they make you feel?"

"They make me feel very happy for them."

"Do they make you think about—?" She stopped midstride. I passed her and then turned back. She wiggled her brows.

"Marriage?" I asked.

"No, silly. Will-B."

"Mother."

"Mother, what? Don't pretend that part of you doesn't wish you were with him today."

"I don't," I shrieked. I hadn't told her about the email, but my mother's motives were clear: she wanted to match-make me right back to Kentucky.

"The lady doth protest too much," she shouted, laughing and slapping me on the back.

Suppressing my smile, I padded up the stairs behind my mother and followed her through a hallway, fragrant with the sea breeze and the perfume emanating from the ladies in swishy workout suits. Past a bin of sheets, Mom swiped the door with her card and opened it to a crisp white bedroom with a tightly made bed and a window—overlooking, yes, the newlyweds.

I dressed for my next appointment—with the grief specialist Ava Torre-Bueno—thinking how I had had a safe and legal procedure, an ostensible "choice." But the two women had not had any choice but to die, risk death, or be killed. I asked my foremothers—Kate Morgan and the woman from Room 3502—for permission to grieve. Then I hit the road for my session with Ava. I wanted to learn how to grieve without spinning out in a vortex of shame.

IN THE WEEKS LEADING UP TO this meeting, I had taken a journey on the Internet to trace the history of abortion around the world, how terminations were done before *Roe v. Wade* made them legal in the United States in 1973, and what motivated Ava to counsel clients who had ended a pregnancy. I hunted down every gem I could find, all from behind my office desk.

People had been having abortions since ancient times in Greece, the Roman Republic, China, Egypt, and the Persian Empire. Between 2737 and 2696 BCE, a Chinese emperor named Shen Nung penned medical texts about it. Plato and Aristotle supported it. The Ebers Papyrus of Egypt, dated to circa 1550 BCE, made reference to abortion. The Hippocratic Oath, which emerged around 400 BCE, ordered physicians to avoid a certain abortion method that would harm a woman. A textbook containing a Persian doctor's instructions for the procedure was published in the tenth century.

I found such comfort in the knowledge that having an abortion wasn't a new human phenomenon, like cell phones and Internet porn. Our bodies had been carrying and releasing children when Jesus walked the earth—and even thousands of years beforehand. Women hadn't always been the ones writing the history, but at least the medical records could show me what I suspected all along: that I had taken my place behind a long line of female ancestors, most of them ghosts by now, who would understand the pain, fear, love, and strength of ending a pregnancy.

To my surprise, there was a time when abortion was neither legal nor illegal in the United States: the procedure was outlawed in 1867 (and remained illegal until 1973). Before 1867, midwives—women healers, who were the respected medical providers before the authorities dubbed them "witches"—traveled from house to house to assist with birth and to prescribe herbal remedies. Black women in slavery exchanged stories and recipes so that women had the power to choose not to carry pregnancies against their will. Then, the American Medical Association advocated for the criminalization of abortion, seeking to disempower female medical healers and to transfer the power to the hands of the then-all-male membership.

During the Victorian Age in the United States and England, print ads surreptitiously advertised abortifacients: "Preventative Powders for married ladies" and "treatment of obstinate case of female irregularity." Women used branded medicines, too, such as a laxative called Beecham's Pills. New York City's Madam Restell (alias of Ann Trow Lohman) was a famous nineteenth-century abortionist who lived in a swanky apartment on Fifth Avenue and had an impressive criminal record for her abortion provisions. From 1938 to the 1950s, the Detroit-based physician Dr. Edgar Bass Keemer Jr. performed procedures for black women, regardless of their incomes. Women also had abortions blindfolded to protect the anonymity of their doctors, who were breaking the law. The inventory of DIY techniques used at home could take up pages: swallowing acid, cottonseed oil, quinine and chloroquine, turpentine, bleach; black market herbs; pounding the belly with a pestle; inserting a bicycle spoke, clothes hangers, a knitting needle, leeches (blood-sucking worms), or a lump of sugar.

Next, I read Ava's story. In 1962, when she was ten years old, her mother was rushed to the hospital from their home in a Sicilian neighborhood of Astoria, Queens. Her father and older brother offered no explanation, so she feared her mother was dead. After a long and unbearable week, a neighbor mentioned to Ava that her mother would be coming home soon. And she did—with a crushing depression.

Ava's parents' birth control had failed, resulting in an unplanned pregnancy. Already scrimping by, the couple could not afford to raise a third child. Her mother, Evelyn, was introduced to a gynecologist who was willing to perform a safe and illegal procedure. It was fairly common for doctors to provide underground services, but they typically charged at least $1,000 (and bargained for sex in some cases) because no laws existed to regulate this covert practice.

The precise number of illegal abortions can never be determined with certainty. Most of them occurred in secret. Forensic pathologists weren't usually trained to identify the signs of such a procedure: this meant that the cause of death went unrecorded for some fatal abortions. The number of unlawful abortions before 1973 is estimated to have ranged from 200,000 to 1.2 million per year, compared with today's rate of approximately 1.06 million. An estimated five thousand women died of unsafe and illegal abortions each year before *Roe.*

The doctor asked Ava's mother for $1,000 for the procedure—almost $8,000 in 2016, taking inflation into account. For the Torre-Buenos, that may as well have been $1 million. So at sixteen weeks of pregnancy, Evelyn locked herself in the bathroom and inserted a blunt object into her uterus. She aborted a baby boy.

Even though Evelyn had sterilized the object, she went into septic shock and was rushed to the hospital. Doctors knew how to help her because hospitals regularly admitted women for perforations and infections that resulted from illegal abortions. But the wave of depression that followed Evelyn home crashed on Ava and her family, leaving them in chaos. Ava spent a decade of adulthood healing the wounds of her mother's sorrow.

Ava worked for Planned Parenthood of San Diego and Riverside Counties for ten years, five of them as director of counseling. In 1976, at the age of twenty-six, she had begun volunteering to protect women from sidewalk picketers by ushering them into clinics. She also held their hands during the procedure.

I asked Ava on the phone how people felt about their abortions in the 70s, believing I might think less of my own problems, which probably paled in comparison. For them, all too recently, having an abortion had been synonymous with back alleys and blindfolds and black market herbs. They knew reproductive rights were nothing to take for granted. When Ava first volunteered at Planned Parenthood, she told me, the women seldom reported mixed feelings, other than a blend of gratitude and relief. But by the end of 1976, they were telling her, "I know I did something really bad." Ava quizzed them to understand why they assumed she was going to judge them. "All those people are against it," they replied. She watched the culture of shame develop before her eyes.

The abortion war had intensified through late 1976, when conservative activists began drumming up support to pass the Hyde Amendment, which would deny financial support for the procedure to federal prisoners, Medicaid recipients, military personnel, and Peace Corps volunteers, except to protect the life of the pregnant person. Picketers gathered outside clinics with their placards.

"They traumatized our patients," Ava said. "The Anti's talk about abortion being traumatic. And it can be. But the clients I've seen who had real posttraumatic stress disorder had it from walking past people waving giant signs in their faces and screaming 'baby killer.' *That* was the trauma that needed to be undone. The Anti's harm women. They keep women in distress."

Colleagues urged her to write a book, but it seemed traitorous for a Planned Parenthood veteran like Ava to acknowledge that some people suffer after abortion. Nonetheless, Ava had credibility as a reproductive freedom activist: she had organized the local chapter of the National Abortion Rights Action League. Her mother had experienced a bad spell of depression after an illegal abortion. Ava had counseled thousands of women at Planned Parenthood, and also men, who felt grief, guilt, anger, regret, and sadness. Her history seemed to relieve the politically constructed tension between rights and recovery.

"I'm not a writer," she said to her colleagues. "Someone else should do this."

But she did do it. Ava published *Peace After Abortion* in 1996. The revised edition is a teal blue paperback. The cover is a picture of a full moon hanging over a forest of bare winter trees.

"Women have more emotional and spiritual pain after abortion than the current research suggests," she declares in the introduction. "I can be supportive of every woman's right to make her own pregnancy decisions, and still recognize the fact that her decision may cause her tremendous suffering."

After risking her professional reputation to publish her book, Ava faced instant blowback—from pro-choicers. She asked the Executive Director of an Insanely Powerful and Famous and Well-Funded Reproductive Health Organization (who shall remain nameless at Ava's request) to throw a book party to drop the paperback into the laps of the people who needed it. "You're just a dupe for the Anti's," he snapped, "and no, you can't have that party with us."

Then Ava took her book to a family reunion. Her aunt had illegally terminated a pregnancy in the 1940s, during the reproductive rights prohibition, and felt extremely uncomfortable that her niece had penned a book that validated grief, guilt, shame, and spiritual injury.

Her aunt said, "*I never had any lingering doubts.*"

"You and plenty of other women," Ava replied, always quick to dispel the assumption that anyone should feel obliged to feel certain emotions. Supporting people who wanted to heal after an abortion was her objective—significantly, without asking them to condemn their own decision as a compulsory stage in recovery.

Ava pedaled the book as a one-woman show, selling one thousand copies by word of mouth. Health clinics, psychologists, and general readers snapped up every last one. She had to run a second printing.

I SAT IN THE CAR OUTSIDE the tall office building of Ava's private counseling practice in San Diego, flipping through *Peace After Abortion.* I recognized similarities between the psychotherapeutic philosophy of Ava and that of Theresa Burke, the founder of Rachel's Vineyard. Both named grief, guilt, depression, anger, and spiritual injury as common emotions. Both acknowledged that men, too: can experience this as a loss. But there are also differences in their interpretations. According to Theresa Burke, people who have had an abortion lash out at picketers because preexisting "trauma" from the termination itself is "being triggered," and so they "attack the messenger because they can't process the message." According to Ava, picketers cause most of the psychological harm she has treated.

AVA WELCOMED ME INTO HER OFFICE. Her salt and pepper hair was pulled back into a loose ponytail. Silver bracelets were stacked up her wrists. She wore a purple skirt and a red shirt with birds flying across it.

More than a decade earlier, Ava had told me, she was driving home after giving a lecture and she burst into tears. She pulled over on the highway, overwhelmed with grief over her brother who had never been born. She was thirty-eight at the time. When she finished crying, she pulled back onto the highway and continued to sit with people like me. I already trusted her.

She motioned for me to take a seat on the couch. I cozied up with her book in my lap, sixteen years after it had first been published.

"How does your abortion come up in a problematic way for you?" Ava asked me with a relaxed, soothing, direct tone of voice. She squared up to me in her office chair.

"It's a constant nagging sensation," I told her.

"Your heart is not at ease," Ava said.

Five years of sobriety had made me raw and sensitive. When I was drinking, I was too cool to be sad. Now I was too sober not to be. "This will sound dramatic," I continued, "but I feel I will never become the person I want to become if I don't do all the emotional and spiritual work it takes to heal around my abortion. The problem is, I don't know *how* to do the work. I need tools."

Ava punctuated her speech with careful gestures and the occasional jazz hands. "I think the problem is, you have had a loss. You are afraid to grieve, so it keeps creeping up on you."

I loved that it wasn't a medical diagnosis; it was a human experience: ungrieved grief.

"Grieving is scary," I said, "especially when so many people don't get it—like most people talking about abortion in public. So far, I've heard two options: grieve your heart out, and then sign this affidavit to try and overturn Roe"—I was referring to the pack of legal documents distributed at Rachel's Vineyard—"*or* don't grieve at all for a first-trimester pregnancy termination in college that allowed you to pursue your education, career goals, and personal freedom."

"Well, with my nearly forty years of experience in this field, I'm here to tell you, some women have real difficulty after this procedure, and it's *our* responsibility to take care of them," Ava said.

All cultures had a version of the Grief Cops, Ava explained. They enforced what grief should look like—grief over any loss—and how long it ought to last. Often, the rules applied specifically to women. Egyptian culture expected women to howl and convulse until they went limp. Balinese culture expected women to maintain composure to avoid making other people feel sad. In America, a person who has an abortion is expected either to grieve with contrition or to act like it was no big deal.

"Ugh. F*ck the Grief Police," I said, already dabbing my eyes with a tissue. Grieving was spilling my holy guts to God, and hell if anybody was going to tell me how to talk to God.

"That's right," Ava said. "Recognizing dogma as the enemy can be very liberating."

She didn't mean the dogma of just the Grief Police. She meant my own dogma, too.

Ava broke down what appeared to be a crisis of grief in the United States, where, it turns out, grieving is almost as taboo as abortion. We have very few models for grief and mourning in this country, Ava said. We have no education in loss. The last image of public mourning in the United States that Ava could recall was Jackie Kennedy wearing a black veil on her pillbox hat in 1963 after JFK's assassination.

Grief is the emotional, physical, and spiritual process by which one experiences a loss—any loss. "Mourning" means practicing the rituals that represent or induce grief. Attending a funeral (mourning) may cause tears (grief). I define mourning as the creative expression of grief, sometimes by a social or religious tradition, such as attending a funeral Mass or making a casserole, and sometimes by improvisation, such as creating a home altar with photographs, heirlooms, candles, and icons of Jesus, Buddha, and Dolly Parton.

Wearing black signifies a spiritual death. During the Victorian Age, women dressed in black crepe dresses and jewelry made of jet, which was sometimes braided with the hair of the departed. Women wept on graves, posing for photographers. Ava told me these communities recognized people as mourners. In the Greco-Roman world, professional mourners were hired to weep. Respect for loss was woven into the fabric of society. And it still was, in other countries.

"Jews wail and rend their clothes," Ava told me. "Arabs wail and hit themselves. They do this now."

Ava reached over and beat her back with one fist. I wanted to do the same, but instead I folded my hands in my lap. Dread slithered down my arms and legs. I told her I didn't want to regress and have another crack-up like the one I had experienced at Rachel's Vineyard. The one where I cried so hard I could barely say the word "toughie."

Spiritual fitness is similar to physical fitness: mindset is everything, approach is everything, technique is everything. True for meditation. True for prayer. True, I suspected, for grief as well. There is a period of time after an overwhelming loss when grief is a volatile animal that can't be tamed. When the power of choice returns, you can run from grief or you can consciously walk through the tunnel toward the little light in the distance. I ran for six years. I had even tried to bypass grief with meditation, sitting at the opening of the tunnel in the lotus position. Now I was game to start walking—or keep walking, as it were.

"The point isn't that we should rend our clothes and beat ourselves," Ava continued, talking with her hands in the air like she was holding a medicine ball. "The point is, because we live in a grief-negative culture, which has moved too far away from acknowledgment of and support for mourners, we all have ungrieved grief. If you begin actively grieving in front of someone else, they have to go *Smack!* because you're stirring up their unconscious grief! After you have experienced a loss—a pregnancy or any other—they'll say to you, 'You look so good.' Subtext: Don't let me see you looking sad. Subtext: you're bringing up my own ungrieved grief. Or, six months after someone loses a spouse of twenty years, people say, 'Are you dating yet?' Grieving a long-term spouse is a two- to five-year process. No less. The subtext of all this is: I don't want to know about your grief, because it freaks me out with all my ungrieved business."

I scooted to the edge of the couch. "It's like when people say, 'You weren't ready to have a baby.' Or, 'Why didn't you choose adoption?' Or, my personal favorite, 'I don't support what you did, but I support you.' Even the remarks that *sound* like support can shut down the conversation: 'I support your right to choose.' That person is sending the message 'Don't grieve around me.'"

It seemed to me that all of America would have ungrieved grief around abortion, from the thousands of people who died before 1973 because of illegal terminations to the people like me who felt the loss of a pregnancy.

Forbidden grief is everywhere, not just in the world of pregnancy. There is plenty of cultural validation for the idea that sorrow is something to fear. Funerals have been replaced with "Celebrations of Life." *The Diagnostic and Statistical Manual of Mental Disorders* (DSM-5) added a so-called problem called "complicated grief disorder," which applied to grief lasting longer than six months, diagnosed using an inventory of symptoms. I thought that The Harebrained Idea That a Griever Ought to Finish Up in a Prescribed Time Frame Lasting No Longer Than Six Months should be added to DSM-6. My country-men seemed staunchly committed to bypassing natural emotions by every available means, and so did I.

"How long do you think the grieving will take me?" I asked Ava.

"It depends on how committed you are to finishing. Instead of grieving all the way through, some people jump off the line," Ava told me. "We jump off into alcohol, or drugs, or food, or movies, or grad-uate school, or work. We spend lifetimes not grieving"—she paused and we met eyes—"What do you think grief looks like?"

"When I jog in the park, I notice the children on swing sets and wonder what mine would have looked like. Creepy, I know."

"It's not that creepy. But it's not grieving, either," Ava said. "Imagining an alternative life with a baby you didn't have is *avoiding* grief. So when you notice your mind going there, just gently remind yourself: 'But I did not have a baby. I had an abortion.'" She told me that this reminder would help deliver me back to reality.

"Ava, where have you been all my life? Why could I only find therapists for issues like videogame addiction and 'moving to NYC,' but not pregnancy termination?"

"Most therapists aren't trained to talk about abortion," she said. That was, almost verbatim, what Dr. Lou, her ideological opponent, had pointed out at Rachel's Vineyard. This underground society of healers could be the realm where the abortion war, as we know it, comes to an end. Peace, love, and therapists.

The crash course in grief continued. "All choice involves loss," Ava said. We carry all sorts of griefs, not just the deaths of loved ones. Leaving a crummy job for a sexy new career is a loss. Marriage is a loss of loves not chosen, as well as a loss of singlehood and independence. With some choices, the alternative remains a mystery: one college over another, abortion over a child.

Which brought me to a perplexing question: "How do I grieve a person I have never met?" How do you grieve a thing that never happened?

Ava's answer was awesomely practical: she suggested that I choose an object to represent the loss and decide for myself what was "lost." The object could be a feather, a marble egg, a photograph.

"But I'm afraid I'm going to regret my decision if I keep grieving."

At Rachel's Vineyard, several alumni told us their regret was unshakable; I'd assumed that's what the end of grief looked like.

"Regret is a defense *against* grieving," said Ava. "We regret so that we don't have to grieve."

"You're blowing my mind," I said. "Because I'm afraid I'll reach the place where I won't be able to accept what happened."

Ava shook her head no. "Grief is the process of coming to acceptance." She pressed her palms together and lowered her voice. "Listen," she said. "If you cried, if you really sobbed for forty minutes, what would happen next?"

"I'd probably eat a loaf of bread and pass out."

"Right. Because sobbing is hugely physical. You'll also be finished with part of the grieving process. Do you know the grief myth? It goes like this: if I go in there, I will never come out. People imagine that when they grieve, they fall down this dark, steep-sided pit. The true image is the long, dark tunnel with openings on both ends. It's full of pain. You keep going. Agony. Grief is agony. You keep going. You reach a real resolution of the loss. Grief is an incredible gift, but you have to have experienced it once all the way through to know the myth isn't true. People say wisdom comes with age. Pfft! No. Wisdom comes with what age gives you the opportunity to do, which is to grieve."

"So how do I begin to grieve?" I asked, clutching my damp tissue.

"Start with thirty seconds," Ava said. "No distractions. No meditating. No thinking. What might help you is imagery. Imagine, as you're starting to grieve, that you're taking a protector with you. A tiger, an angel, an animal. Doesn't matter. Let yourself feel what comes up. Try to tolerate it for thirty seconds."

"I will try," I said. I was afraid. Very. But this was a lesson I had to learn again and again: faith comes after I do what scares me, not before. I had to be afraid and grieve anyway.

- 11 -

HOW TO TAKE UP SPACE

SIX YEARS, TWO MONTHS, AND ONE WEEK AFTERWARD—I wrapped my hands around the steering wheel, speeding north to Santa Barbara, where my evening with Terra Wise, the Midwife for the Soul, would begin at nightfall. Mom sat quietly in the passenger's seat. The windows were down, the car hummed, and the air smelled like cocoa butter, fish, rubber, and salt. As the lane narrowed and wound along the edge of the sand, I started feeling like a fraud, moving on to the next expert before I'd even tried thirty seconds of grief. But Mom beat me to it. When I turned up the radio, a Motown station, breaking the silence, she reached for the knob and turned it back down.

"You know, Kass, we've lived miles apart for so long," she said. "Sometimes I feel like I don't even know you."

"We talk on the phone every day," I reminded her, aware that it was a tepid consolation.

"You don't know it yet, but nobody else will ever listen to you like your mother listens to you. I could call my mom saying I broke a nail, and five minutes later, she'd be sitting on my couch. She'd frame a napkin that I sneezed in." Her voice went wobbly. "Damn," she said, lying back in the seat. "What's wrong with me?"

"Nothing is," I said. I told her I missed her mother, too. She turned toward the window, away from me, to dab the corners of her eyes. She tugged a crumpled tissue out of her purse—it was smudged with buff powder and lord knows what else.

"Well, anyway, I just wish we'd see more of each other."

I suggested we video chat.

"You bond with someone through shared experience," she said.

"Isn't this a shared experience?"

She laughed. "Touché," she said, dabbing her eye again.

"Remember Orlando?" she asked.

Orlando. When I was fifteen years old, I decided to get serious about becoming a runway model. This dream was unlikely to come true, given my five-foot-five stature and the inbreeding that could be seen in my eyes. My great-grandparents were first cousins.

The path that led from Kentucky to the runway began at a local modeling agency called Vogue to which the modeling hopeful would pay an absurdly high fee to be groomed for an absurdly expensive conference wherein she may or may not get scouted by a career-level agency. My mother cobbled together the money to send me to Vogue.

It was there in a strip mall office wallpapered in headshots that I learned how to eat half a banana for lunch and create a "signature" runway walk.

At the end of the summer, our group of Kentucky models headed down to Orlando to be scouted. I had spent the summer smoking marijuana and eating entire bananas and worse: sandwiches. I stood in the foyer of the conference center with my mother, feeling like we were two dogs at a horse show. Leggy models zipped by, gaps between their thighs that would drop a softball.

"Don't compare yourself," my mother said, sensing my apprehension.

"Don't worry," I said. "There's no comparison."

Our first stop was the Urgent Treatment Center. I had twisted my ankle in a drunken tumble the night before and simultaneously came down with a case of strep throat that was causing my voice to frog out. Within minutes of popping the first pill, a relief map of welts appeared on my skin. That's when I discovered I was allergic to opiates, I clawed at the hives on my arms, legs, chest, and neck.

"Mama, why?"

She gazed pitifully at my breakout. "I think this is just God's way of telling us that this isn't your path," she replied.

The next morning, I wiggled into a yellow floral one-piece bathing suit that my mother and I had picked out in a department store in Kentucky. When the announcer called my name, I did my best sauntering hobble onto the catwalk, leading with a beer gut. The crowd was packed in the thousands and the lights were so hot that beads of sweat rolled down my hive-splotched back as I completed my turn to the sound of half-hearted applause.

That night while I slept hard because of antihistamines, my mother stayed up waiting for my callback. Around 2 A.M., the phone rang. It was the director of Vogue expressing his condolences that none of the agencies was interested in my look. I hadn't tried hard enough to warrant feeling like a failure, but I did feel ugly.

The next day, my mother took me to Disney World. We wore giant Mickey Mouse ears and gorged on pastel-colored cakes. We pulled pink cotton candy from a cone and spun around on the teacups. We traipsed all over the place, taking turns doing impressions of my "signature" runway walk. I swayed my hips from side to side, dipping low with every other step. "No, no," my mother said. "It's like this." She imitated me, adding an exaggerated frown.

"It was money well spent," my mother said as I exited toward Santa Barbara. She had her arms crossed over her pastel windbreaker.

"Three thousand dollars? So I could limp down a runway looking like a pimple?"

I shifted in my seat, one hand on the wheel.

"You had been so content to earn C's for years in school. It made me furious because I knew you were smart. I called you the Queen of C."

"I don't remember you calling me that," I said.

"You never listened. It was money well spent because you realized that modeling was a pipe dream. And it was a hollow dream. You were going to have to do something with your brain if you wanted to make it in this world."

"Or get a chin job."

"You made the right choice. You were meant to be a writer and a teacher. I wanted to be a writer, too, you know."

"I know."

"I wanted to be like Erma Bombeck. I had this romantic idea that I'd go write books in the mountains. My mother told me to get my teaching degree to fall back on. I fell back on it for thirty years."

"What do you think stopped you from writing?"

"Marriage. Kids. A sixty-five-hour workweek. Life goes by in a blink. One day you're suddenly divorced and remarried and retired and your kids are grown up and you remember that you used to have dreams of your own."

ONE WAY TO SUMMARIZE MY NIGHT in a motel with Terra Wise is to tell you that I acted like a bitch and then she gave me the best free medicine there is. She asked what my heart felt and I replied with existential one-word answers, like "nothing." She tried to teach me that a proper breathing technique would help me commune with the muscle of radiance in my rib cage, and I commented that I hadn't budgeted for a lesson in breathing given that air is free of charge and this session was not.

Terra had been an international educator since 1983. She led workshops and seminars on womb loss, breath work, and somatic therapy, among other areas of expertise. "My work helps people cross thresholds," she told me, in my case, the threshold from head to heart. There was a time when I would have cackled at such an anti-intellectual concept. And I sort of did, at first. But dropping into my heart rivaled getting sober in terms of difficulty. Most of her clients were women, plus couples and men, too, who had undergone one or more abortions. "All people deserve respect and compassion and an opportunity to work through unresolved feelings after abortion," she said. According to her website, her Womb Wisdom™ offered "support and guidance in the days, months, and even decades after abortion."

Canadian by birth, Terra just happened to be cruising through California when I needed her. Hence the motel room. The headboard was made of faux leather and matched the rest of the room's kitschy accessories, all upholstered in the same blackish purple fabric: the two bucket chairs by the windows, the frame around the mirror. Even the tissue box looked like a bruise.

When I'd booked the appointment with Terra over the phone, I had asked her what a session with "The Midwife for the Soul" was supposed to do. "This work creates feelings of freedom and choice. It will feel as if you 'push out' the things that block your path and your goals," she told me, "I will help you to birth the best parts of yourself."

So far that meant lying on my back on the bed with Terra kneeling over me, clutching my bare foot and commanding me to push into her hands.

She resembled Sandra Bullock, had a silver stud in her nose. Fifty-two years old, she had skin so smooth it looked airbrushed. She had the body of a dancer—lithe, graceful—and hair like a black flame. I felt a black flame inside my head, as if the ungrieved grief had turned my brain into a burning stress center.

"Why do I need to push into your hands?" I asked.

"I'm trying to exhaust the muscle tension in your body," she said, with a smooth Elizabeth Hurley cadence. "Your energy is up in your head. You're disassociating from the pain, Miss I'm-Okay-I'm-Fine-I'm-Just-Doing-Analysis. There is something inside you, but you're holding back. And that's fine. We can do shallow work. You'll still pay me for the session, but we don't have to go in all the way."

"I want to go in all the way," I interrupted her, kicking her hands as hard as I could.

This exercise is called "Somatic experiencing." *Soma* means body, as opposed to mind. In *Waking the Tiger: Healing Trauma: The Innate Capacity to Transform Overwhelming Experiences,* medical biophysicist and psychologist Dr. Peter Levine explains that elements of an overwhelming experience freeze inside the body and must be re-integrated into the authentic self. The frozen parts stay stuck until a person returns awareness to the body and "thaws" them out.

The goal of the session was for me to defrost my emotions and unshrink my body. This meant learning how to breathe into my belly like a newborn baby. A newborn baby hasn't yet conditioned themselves to fit in. A newborn baby isn't looking for approval. Breathing into the belly, inhaling into the diaphragm, can stir up emotions. Babies cry and laugh and scream and don't care who they make uncomfortable. Somewhere along the line, I had begun pulling shallow gulps of air into my chest. I had a quarter century's worth of toxic messages in my head, messages that tell girls and women to be either small and quiet or small and loud. Messages that tell girls and women not to breathe. According to the patriarchy, women should be thin and demure if they want to be loved. I wanted to be loved and so I got quiet and breathed into my chest instead of my belly because I did not want to look fat. According to certain dogmatic feminists, the only empowered emotion a woman should show is anger. Otherwise, they seemed to say, suck it up and be stoic and over it. When I was twenty-two and at an appointment for an IUD placement, a T-shaped piece of copper was being primitively pushed into my uterus, without so much as an Advil. I whimpered to the nurse: "May I scream?" She was wearing a Rosie the Riveter pin on her scrubs. She got up in my face, nose-to-nose, and said, "No. You can be a woman." Be a woman: bottle up your feelings. Be a woman: be a robot. Do not disturb the emotions. I wanted to be "a woman" and so I took shallow breaths into my chest and swallowed my scream. "Be a woman" means shut up and stay up in your head so people will take you seriously.

I breathed badly for the patriarchy. I breathed badly for toxic breeds of feminism. I "froze" my intense emotions and stored them in my body and tried never to disturb them. I played along because I had no mind of my own while some movements within feminism had, in its effort to expand opportunities for women, degraded the feminine genius of silence, relationships, and love. The skeleton in my closet was never my abortion—it was my heart.

Terra set my foot on the bed and placed her hands over my "womb." "Take a breath, all the way up to your heart. I'm going to breathe with you, and I'm going to make some sounds, and you're going to make them with me. Say AHHHHHHHHH-GAHHHHHHHHH."

She had to be kidding me. I stared at her without blinking.

Terra assured me it was a common somatic healing sound to help release trauma and tension.

"AHHHHHHHH-GAHHHHH," we said together.

"How did you lose the baby?" Terra asked.

"I rejected it," I said, as if speaking on autopilot.

"Can you say more?"

"It was the solution that would get my mother off my back."

Poor Mom. She offers me a place at home during the most humiliating phone call of my life and then I claimed to have rejected motherhood to "get my mother off my back." I wanted my life to belong to me, which meant I wanted my body to belong to me, which meant I had to spread my legs in a most undignified position and pay a doctor to vacate one childhood dream so that I could chase after the dream of setting up my own distinct life. Fast forward six years, though, and I had traveled hundreds of miles away from her, only to follow the red line on her professional map. Like legions of other women, I had become my mother—and I did it by choosing not to become a mother. As it turned out, neither my mother nor my baby (nor even the patriarchy) had been my greatest threats to freedom. My greatest threat to freedom was fear.

Terra slid her hands between the bed and my back, under the wing bones, and instructed me to breathe into her hands. "It's like you're wearing an invisible straitjacket," she said. "You limit how deeply you breathe. When you breathe in and breathe out, when your body actually moves, that's where the emotions can come and go."

Walling off grief was a full-body effort involving my head, my heart, and my lungs. Breathing deeply, in through the nose and out through the mouth, plunked me down into my heart. This is where grief and God came together for me: the English word *spirit* comes from the Latin word *spiritus*. *Spiritus* means *breath*. I experienced God as the present moment. Breathing brought me back to the moment: it required focused attention, on and off the meditation cushion.

"There's a fear that if you breathe you'll be seen," Terra said, removing her hands from under my back and sitting back on her heels. "It keeps you very small. You hold your breath to be invisible. And yet, your deepest desire is to be seen."

I held my breath and wore neon clothes. I held my breath and talked about my abortion with strangers. I held my breath and wanted a flashing Times Square billboard with my ten-foot name and gigantic face, for no apparent reason or merit except to be all over everything, to cover the whole world with myself. I was the tree falling in the woods: if I was alive and nobody saw or heard me, did I still exist?

I was now silently obeying Terra's commands. "Imagine that your breath is like the ocean down the street—and breathe all the way up your body from your toes to your face. Fill your womb. Fill your entire body with the breath."

I inhaled the imaginary sea, pulling water up to the crown of my head.

"Take up room!" Terra cheered. "There ya go, thereyago, thereyago, thereyago. Keep going, keepgoing, keepgoing, keepgoing. That's it, that's it, that's it, that's it. TAKE UP SOME F*CKING SPACE!"

My session with Terra answered three questions with one word.

How do you begin to grieve?

How do you get instant access to God?

How do you take up space?

Breathe.

Suck air. Expand.

In order to take up space, I had to close my mouth. Taking up space doesn't necessarily mean being rowdy and opinionated and irreverent, as though I had to fight for room, because space isn't scarce. Taking up space means knowing the space is mine and being so in touch with the breath that I make room for others to take up space with me.

BACK OUT IN THE PARKING LOT, I found my mother sleeping in the front seat with the seat rolled back, wearing a headband and ponytail. Awakening, she asked, "Well, did that smack of con-artistry?" She didn't expect me to answer.

- 12 -

ANOTHER UNDERGROUND MOVEMENT

SIX YEARS, TWO MONTHS, AND TEN DAYS AFTERWARD—At a Holiday Inn in San Francisco. Six A.M. I swept the shower curtain over to the side and sat on the edge of the tub in baggy sweatpants, my bare feet shoulder width apart. Then I made the mistake of looking in the mirror. My bloodshot eyes looked freakishly green. Dark circles, face sagging in misery. I wanted to go back to sleep. Scratch that. I wanted to go back to my own apartment in Manhattan and lock my bedroom door and shut out every single human being so that I could let these gruesome emotions funnel through me.

My mother was sleeping now, but during the day, she'd taken to strolling up and down the boardwalks, arms swinging, in a white windbreaker embroidered with the words SAN FRANCISCO, carrying a ceramic chocolate-brown mug printed with the word GHIRARDELLI that she had gotten at the factory tour. Now that I had finally dropped from head into heart, the realm I had managed to escape for six years, I was determined to stay out of my personal Thought Center. Unfortunately, my next appointment was scheduled at a placed called a "think tank."

The meeting, an interview with two cutting-edge scholars on how women feel about their abortions, would begin in three hours. I cringed at the thought of buttoning up my stiff blue blazer and masking my pain with firm handshakes and heady academic-speak. But maybe I wouldn't have to. Kate Cockrill ran the Social and Emotional Aspects of Abortion program at a research group called Advancing New Standards in Reproductive Health (ANSIRH) at the University of California, San Francisco. Together with a social movement theorist named Katrina Kimport, she had interviewed dozens of women after their terminations, in order to understand the emotional landscape. Their studies had not been published yet, but I couldn't wait any longer.

Reading published research had saved me when I was pregnant. Only one person in the whole world had ever told me that she'd had an abortion, but the research told me one in three American women would terminate a pregnancy in her lifetime. High statistical likelihood that I'd bump into one or two people who'd had an abortion if I kept on talking.

In those years, I noticed a subtext to conversations about abortion that bordered on authentic. It went like this: *I hope my talking about being sad about my abortion doesn't make you feel bad about not feeling sad about yours.* We had been taught how to feel. We had been taught how not to feel. In the early days after my abortion, defending and explaining how I felt or didn't feel about my abortion had taken so much mental energy that it took me years to get around to the actual work of tending to my emotions. Engaging with this nonsense was my bad.

Sneaking across the pitch-black bedroom, careful not to wake my mother, I blindly rummaged through my bag of papers and books, waiting for my eyes to adjust to the dark while I pulled out three stapled pages of interview prep.

I had originally intended to ask the scholars for research-backed assurance that I was "normal," but I didn't need statistical assurance that I wasn't the only person who'd needed to recover after an abortion. Ava Torre-Bueno wrote: "many women have more emotional and spiritual pain after abortion than the current research suggests." Therapists sometimes use euphemisms like "women's issues" or "pregnancy loss," to advertise after-abortion support without implying that they think a person "should" need to heal, which is considered a sentiment of the "Antis." (This is how it happened: anti-choice activists used emotional pain to advance their political agenda; pro-choice activists denied that most people had emotional pain related to their abortions. Ergo: advertising counseling or therapy for abortion may come across as antiabortion. Ergo: people who are searching for support have to wade through vague advertising, just to get a dang therapist.) Terra Wise had described her clients as "falling apart," "catatonic," and "literally nuts." A list of Christian psychologists specializing in abortion had been distributed at Rachel's Vineyard, which held one thousand retreats for healing after abortion each year in forty-eight states and fifty-eight countries. Backline was a phone counseling service for reproductive health in the United States and Canada. Exhale, an after-abortion talkline, counseled callers nationwide in six different languages. Numerous religious ministries run after-abortion hotlines, support groups, and retreats, many of them listed through a centralized database at abortionrecovery.org.

Not all people who call these places can't wrangle their feelings. Some people just crave a connection with somebody who gets it. Some people just want to talk about it, or a place to go, or a ritual. Some people might want to name the baby. Doesn't mean they're in shambles—and doesn't mean they're not in shambles, either.

Back in the bathroom, seated on the edge of the tub with papers in my lap. The tip of my pen ripped across the paper as I crossed out my interview questions with a big blue X.

I figured Kate and Katrina must have been well aware that sound bites and attempts to capture us "in a nutshell" or a "syndrome" were ridiculous and impossible, so I had a new question for them, which now seems presumptuous: How *soon* could I expect a study that documents sisterhoods and siblinghoods and revolutions of healing after abortion?

Even though my heart felt like a voodoo doll being stabbed with a thousand tiny needles and I wanted to hide and cry, I was showing up at the meeting, and not just for myself. For Amy, who also had nowhere to go for community after her abortion but a retreat run by protesters who might have screamed "baby killer" as she entered the clinic. I stepped off the elevator in the "think tank." Kate stood up from her desk and reached out to pump my hand. She had fringed brown bangs chopped off mid-forehead, a bright, cautious smile, and the angular face of a younger Frances McDormand, all vaulting brows and bones chiseled sharp.

"Nice boots," she said. Mine were a battered shade of ivory, hers bucolic brown.

Kate introduced me to her colleague, Dr. Katrina Kimport, a qualitative sociologist. She wore a cardigan with a matching shell and had an au naturel look.

We went to a café around the corner where we organized around a table with mugs of coffee in front of us.

"What sparked your interest in reproductive health and emotions?" I asked them both, timidly sipping my coffee from my mug. I already felt small and dumb, like I always felt around ultra-educated and well-spoken women. As soon as I breathed, I lost track of what they were saying, so I inhaled shallow gulps of air and listened.

Kate had volunteered for the National Abortion Federation hotline. Katrina had been reading *Ms.* magazine since the age of twelve. Neither mentioned having had an abortion.

They told me about their as-yet unreleased studies about regret.

"These women we interview don't say, 'I was having a great time and then I walked out of the clinic and everything fell to pieces,'" said Kate, seated across from me. "We're trying to move away from the belief that someone's abortion causes her negative feelings."

I nodded enthusiastically, trying to make this objective okay with me, even though it wasn't.

"Women who've had multiple procedures feel differently about each one," said Katrina, clasping her hands over the table, a wedding band on her finger. "This is evidence that the actual procedure does not cause sadness. The procedure does not pose a risk for sadness."

"Nor does the woman," added Kate.

"Nor does the woman," Katrina said. "Neither the woman nor the procedure is at fault for any sadness that occurs. It's the situation that causes sadness."

I repeated her words: *The situation causes sadness.*

If Rachel's Vineyard zeroed in almost exclusively on the deliberate loss of a "baby" as the cause of all suffering, the scholars fixated almost exclusively on the academic doublespeak of "circumstances." Take the weight off of the abortion and disperse it. A new spin on the same reductive political sound bite I could have heard if I turned on the television.

It felt like they were using language that would trivialize these thoughts and emotions.

Katrina's study on regret was published two years later. In "(Mis)understanding Abortion Regret," she reported that "negative" feelings after abortion occurred for one of three simple reasons: "loss of romantic relationship," "social disapproval," and "head versus heart conflict." All three reasons were valid, all three true for me, but the report was incomplete. Then I found an explanation of the recruitment process for the study with a troubling detail: phone counselors at two secular talklines supporting people after abortion told their callers about the

opportunity to be interviewed. About half of potential study participants couldn't even be invited for an interview because talkline counselors deemed them too distraught—so it had seemed inappropriate
for the counselor to mention an academic study. How could the study
have gone on, when women presenting the strongest emotions after an
abortion could not be invited to participate in a study about emotions
after abortion? Was it possible that some scholars claiming to discover
the communal story about abortion were also shaping it?

I wanted to roar, *you have no* idea *what causes sadness.* Instead, I began
stammering, trying to work up the nerve to ask, *why are we still afraid
to talk about the fact that abortion can have profound emotional and mental
impact on some people? Why did destigmatizing abortion have to mean making it seem painless and simple?*

I also had a subtextual question: *If I tell the truth about my abortion,
the brilliant hilarious defiant women I love will back away slowly, yes? I'm not
in the club anymore, am I?*

"The pro-choice movement has been professionalized," said Kate.

"Exactly," said Katrina. "The movement has organizations that
represent reproductive rights, so people who identify as pro-choice
and suggest that some people are going to have a really tough time
are seen as a chink in the armor of this movement."

I shrunk in my seat and placed my hands gingerly in my lap, swallowing the bitter taste of my own medicine. Six years earlier, I'd drop-
kicked my abortion story into the ears of anybody who would listen,
trying to be a counterpoint to cautionary tales about abortion. I was
on a mission to let everyone know that we had been fed a story about
abortion that wasn't true. It wasn't about "killing babies" or moral
failings or being sad bad women. I said things like: I made the best
decision. No regrets. My body, my choice. Such was the feminist story
that was already out in the world and available for me to tell. It made
me feel like a good feminist to tell it.

But it was ridiculously problematic, that story. What that story didn't say was, the same conservative system that set up so many of us to get pregnant by accident, was the same creepy system that made bringing a child into the world seem like a brutal thing to do. The same system that taught abstinence-only sex education and told girls that our sexuality was dangerous and dirty and the sole source of our value, and gave boys and men no responsibility for their sexual behavior, and taught everyone to grasp somewhere outside themselves for self-esteem, and used religious dogma to erode our connection with divine guidance, was the same system in which I got pregnant. The same system that paid women significantly less than men and refused to guarantee a livable minimum wage and denied paid parental leave and subsidized daycare, was the same system that shook their heads at the scourge of addiction and waged a "War on Drugs" and locked up would-be fathers like Noah and branded them with felony records that followed them for life and made them unemployable, was the same system shaming people for using government assistance to support their families, was the same system that looked down upon teen moms and single moms, particularly if they weren't white and wealthy, was the same system that said abortion was murder and shut down abortion clinics, was the same system that said that our feelings of devastation meant that something was wrong with abortion without admitting that something was wrong with their system.

The "situation" really was everything. And yet, for years after my meeting with the scholars, I fell down countless philosophical rabbit holes trying to figure out why their theory that "the situation" caused sorrow didn't land for me. Their theory seemed unfalsifiable, but it also choked the conversation: It's not the abortion. It's not the woman. So it's definitely not abortion that hurts women. [Subtext: stop saying that an abortion caused sadness.] It's the situation that causes any sadness. The thing was, "the situation" itself was a trap, and it wasn't all specific to my story. We had a collective story, a collective situation. The Situation. It was the story of girls and women who had always been left alone to fight our way out of traps and then expected to shut up and be grateful that we had a way out at all. When we stopped talking about suffering around abortion, then we stopped talking about why just having a way out wasn't good enough. Talking about the pain gave us hope for doing away with the traps altogether.

What boggled my mind, though, was how Kate and Katrina hadn't interviewed the same people I was meeting, why Kate told me at one point that she thought suffering after an abortion was "rare." Perhaps I hadn't adequately explained what I meant by "suffering." I saw suffering as knowing that something was wrong with the whole experience of getting pregnant and feeling that terminating it is the most loving choice, but not knowing how to articulate what felt so wrong. I saw suffering as the time between having a massively meaningful experience and being able to articulate it. Suffering meant having to hide that I was excited about my pregnancy after it was over—that it was, indeed, the abortion, the fact that it ended without a baby, that allowed me to feel such a thrill about it.

Of course, suffering also meant crying jags and intrusive thoughts and psychic pain. If the women who were too distraught to be included in a study about emotions had been interviewed, what might they have said? Could the truth be told in an academic study? Would I let them have such a sacred story? But I found one reason why certain experiences go undocumented, why the scholars and I didn't see the same reality about abortion.

"What was the Catholic program like?" Kate asked me.

"There were a lot of awkward hugs," I said, suddenly embarrassed about the babies.

"You needed to go to such a place to feel better?" Katrina asked.

Both women listed forward. Kate cupped one ear to hear me over the white noise of the coffee shop.

Admit to being a chink in the armor?

"Oh, no," I lied. "I was basically there as a journalist"—one of those journalists who sobs uncontrollably after naming her aborted baby for one of the twelve tribes of Israel. I didn't want to tell them that I embodied the shadow self of the pro-choice movement. I was also still figuring out my story. The parts I hadn't figured out yet were the parts I hadn't heard anybody talk about, the thoughts and emotions and interactions that hadn't been sucked into the political machine or picked to the bone in academia.

We left our table, slid our coffee mugs across the counter, and filed out onto the sidewalk. Pedestrians in houndstooth blazers and sneakers crisscrossed in front of us carrying to-go coffees.

"I'm coming in for an awkward hug," said Kate. She opened her arms to me.

I DROVE AWAY FROM THE "THINK TANK," envisioning a community where we could come together to recognize abortion as a beginning of spiritual emergence. I wasn't interested in safe topics. I was interested in talk of blood and rage and ferocious mother-grief. Zygotes and babies and secret predilections like obsessions with pregnant bellies. We would honor life and death, grief and suffering, friendships and romance, a love of one's own body, mother wounds and daddy issues, the divine. There would be listening and validation, but no coddling, no insistence that abortion was universally the "right decision" or the "wrong decision." If one of us determined that the wrong decision had been made, then we would embrace this admission as an integral personal acknowledgment of wrongdoing, not an indictment of reproductive rights. Stigma had no power over us. Struggle was not a requirement for membership; having had an abortion was.

I crossed into woodsy neighborhoods with Technicolor houses, determined to find a sister—not a guru—who could grasp viscerally my need for a community of people who talked about their terminations without fronting, without pandering to the political conflict, without whispering, without infantilizing or patronizing recovering people, without being too hard or too soft. Not because I'd achieved this level of enlightenment, but because I was trying. When my head dispatched thoughts that told me to stop being so dramatic about my abortion and just go home, I called upon a wise and queenly higher self to pluck the little me and drop her gently back into my heart. Now I was looking not for a think tank but for a luv tank.

My next stop was breakfast with Aspen Baker, the executive director of Exhale and leader of the pro-voice movement. I had cobbled together a stalkerish dossier based on her defunct blog and various online news articles: she was born on January 22, 1976—the third anniversary of *Roe v. Wade*—in San Diego County, California. Her blog covered mostly her dining adventures. A year and a half earlier, she had eaten a Boboli pizza with bacon. And when she wasn't eating Boboli pizza, she was trying to start a revolution.

Unable to contain my excitement about Aspen, I'd phoned her in advance and asked her to tell me how pro-voice was born. Back in 2000, when she was twenty-four years old, she'd gathered with four friends on a living room floor. Markers and loose-leaf papers were strewn about the rug. This assembly of women became the five founders of Exhale, a phone counseling service created for people who had experienced abortion, by people who had experienced abortion.

Exhale had refused to take a side in the war. They weren't pro-choice; they weren't pro-life. They just weren't fighting. Only one of the five foremothers had never had an abortion. She was also the only founder who was adamant that Exhale be labeled "pro-choice," or else they could be perceived as being apathetic about women dying because of illegal abortions. The other founders insisted on holding space for callers who wanted support without having to pander to a side in the war with language that would be "on message."

Four women, staking a claim on their abortions, outside the war. I dug it. More and more, the word *experience* rang truer than the words *story* or *abortion*. A "story" could get stuck. An "abortion" could be misunderstood. A "termination" was an "ending." An experience was expansive and ongoing, evoking wisdom gathered over the passage of time.

Aspen took on credit card debt to research a curriculum for training phone counselors. She recruited candidates and interviewed volunteers in a hallway. The first phone rang in 2002, three days after the line went live from a small loft in an art deco building in downtown Oakland. A founding board chair named Lisa picked up the call. It was a man. Lisa figured it was Aspen's boyfriend, pranking her. But the caller was a father, asking about how to support his daughter who had recently ended her pregnancy.

Next, Exhale opened a national phone line offering counseling in English, Spanish, Mandarin, Vietnamese, Cantonese, and Tagalog.

It rolled out a line of e-cards. Pictures—of a pale orange leaf floating in water or of reeds blowing against a blue sky—could be matched with messages: "I want you to know that I care about you, and how you are feeling. My thoughts are with you." Only one message was overtly religious: "The promise of God is to be with us through all of life's transitions. God will never leave you or forsake you. May you find comfort in God's constant love. Know that my prayers are with you at this time."

Then the e-cards caught Rush Limbaugh's attention:

Now, this Baker babe, founder and executive director of Exhale [Lim-
baugh exhales], said that she was "unaware of anybody else providing
after-abortion sympathy cards online." How convoluted is this? If you're
going to send a sympathy card to anybody after an abortion, shouldn't it
be the aborted fetus?

More than five thousand abortion e-cards were sent from Exhale's website that week alone. After listening to fifteen thousand people over the phone, Aspen and the Exhale counselors were convinced that media portrayals and political debates were reductive and out of touch with reality. There was no "average" person who had an abortion. Exhale callers included Limbaugh fans, dogmatic liberal feminists, and women who were vehemently antiabortion, even during their own terminations. Christians, Buddhists, Jews, Hindus, Muslims, atheists, agnostics, "nones," pagans, witches, and spiritual wanderers called Exhale.

Aspen, who earned a bachelor's degree in Peace and Conflict Studies at UC Berkeley, expanded her vision beyond the talkline toward a broader mission to bring people together in a space free of political agendas. In 2005, she coined the term *pro-voice.* It was the name of her movement that sought to restart the conversation about abortion by focusing on personal experience. In the past, people had told their stories with a motive to influence listeners that abortion should be legal or illegal, depending on what side of the debate they stood for. The pro-voice way was to talk about abortion to connect with another human being simply for the sake of connecting. Pro-voice was a practice of nonviolence—think Gandhi—that emphasized listening and storytelling. If the battlefield mentality dominating the public dialogue about abortion had separated human beings into warring factions, Aspen wanted to bring folks together in friendship and solidarity. Not fully comprehending the scattered nature of social movements, I expected the pro-voice crusade to be marching down the streets of Oakland.

I waited for Aspen on a stool at the smudged window of the Lakeshore Café. A woman crossed the frame, nearly six feet tall with an ash blonde ponytail. Her. The door jingled open. I slid off my stool and glided toward her. I couldn't possibly hug her, could I? It would be too soon.

I couldn't stop myself.

"Hey player," she said.

"Girl. I am so glad this is finally happening."

We slid into a booth along the wall. Aspen had blue eyes, one of which reminded me of a brown-speckled robin's egg. A waitress with silver hoops in her eyebrow, lip, and left nostril took our orders. Aspen ordered a bagel with lox; staying true to my vegan diet, I ordered huevos rancheros, hold the huevos.

We sipped coffee and Aspen told me about her pregnancy. A decade earlier, she was twenty-three and dating a bad boy surfer whom an uncle-ish family friend had warned her to stay away from. Born in a trailer to a Christian surfer family in Orange County, Aspen believed God was love and abortion was "killing." She missed her period. She lined up five home pregnancy tests on the bathroom counter with two blue lines in each miniature window. She thought she was going to become a mother. *Single mother,* her boyfriend clarified. His reaction surprised her—she didn't mind the idea of being a broke parent (she was a waitress), but she hadn't planned on being a single parent.

Given the legal and biological time constraints, she went ahead and scheduled an abortion at a hospital two blocks from her apartment. Insurance would cover it. Aspen was comforted by the knowledge that she could change her mind at the last minute and have the baby; a friend of hers was alive today because her mother had done that. But Aspen didn't.

In the weeks after the procedure, Aspen told me, she started to wrestle with self-respect. She wasn't sure the decision had matched her values. She was shocked that the medical process hadn't involved an element of emotional care. So she booked a private therapist and came to perceive her abortion as "a door" to deeper healing.

A theme was emerging for me. So far on my journey, everybody who knew anything about recovery understood that the termination was the trailhead, the threshold, the portal, the opening to a tunnel. The building manager in a karate uniform at the Buddhist Church had opened the door to a world that was saving me—and had been saving me long before I gave it credit. And it was my abortion that had led me to the door.

I dreaded the end of breakfast. I was flying back to Manhattan the next day. I confessed that I hadn't yet found an abortion posse. The voices on Exhale's talkline were still disembodied. I couldn't make eye contact over the phone or reach across a table and touch people or sit next to them on the couch and look at them. What I really wanted hadn't changed: a sisterhood, a siblinghood, who'd ended pregnancies and then followed the path of the spiritual polestar.

"Where do I find, like, a community?" I asked Aspen. I felt mildly like I was asking her how to make friends, which was perhaps true in some respect. What I meant was, tell me somebody has already created this space, and I can just slip in through the back door and take an inconspicuous seat in the corner of the room and casually make friends and pretend I do not need them like oxygen. Tell me I won't have to own my wanting. Tell me I can satisfy my need without bothering anybody or making a big deal about my pain.

Like many girls, I was taught to tame my wanting. I was called selfish and demanding when I wanted something for myself and weak when what I wanted was help. So I learned to hide my wanting, including my desire to connect with other women, which was the most threatening desire of all. Because women who have had an abortion have seen beneath the surface. Many know secrets about the world that nobody talks about, like that having an abortion is a wilderness, that we will actually kill in order to protect ourselves and our cubs, that the world is not safe for our bodies and our children. Our pain after abortion is so dangerous to the established order that men tried to diagnose it and "explain" our pain to us. They used our pain as evidence for an argument that we needed to be protected from our own agency, that we needed to be controlled for our own good and the good of our children. If we listened to our pain and realized the world had buried us alive and then kicked our way out of the grave, if we heard what our pain wanted and followed its commands, then those men would be in serious motherf*cking trouble.

But desire terrified me with its power and so I medicated it. Alcohol deluged me with the courage to want the things I wasn't supposed to want, like zipless sex and White Castle hamburgers and no shoes and no baby. Now I medicated my desires with Zoloft, with Buddhism ("desire is suffering"), and with my selective silence—talking about my abortion, but not talking about how badly I had wanted it, and how badly I wanted the baby, and how badly I wanted something else, too. Something was wrong, and not just with me. Something was wrong with the world.

"Tell your story," Aspen said, with a tone that was like, *What are you waiting for?!*

Again? I thought, though I sheepishly said, "Okay. I will."

Then her words fell through my head and twirled down like helicopter seeds until they landed. I had to take up some f*cking space. Because a woman who uses her voice to discuss her feelings about her abortion violates every rule: the rule that we shouldn't have abortions because we had to be a hypersexualized virgin or a desexualized mother, the rule that if we couldn't or wouldn't be that, if a single childless woman had an abortion, then she had to be easygoing about it. She pursues her career and never complains about the sacrifices she made to get wherever she got and never admits it if the "career" turned out to feel like meaningless plastic.

I knew that telling the story hadn't healed me, but it was never supposed to heal me. My story was supposed to be a flame signal to connect me with other human beings. What scared me about announcing my need for a community was that groups of honest women tended to expose what I wanted and give my wanting power. Once I told the truth to other women, I couldn't go back into hiding.

AT A VINEYARD IN NAPA VALLEY that evening, I was about to get my mother drunk.

"Late birthday present," I said, handing her a bottle of Cabernet. I was flying back to New York the next day—this was my last shot at a deep talk with her about my abortion. She reached up and threw her arm around my shoulder, pulling me in close until our heads touched and we locked strides.

"My sweet, sweet baby girl," she said. "I appreciate that, Kass."

We carried paper plates of food outside. Mom strutted ahead in paisley clam diggers, her ponytail going thwap-thwap-thwap. We settled into a picnic table on the lawn.

The vineyards looked like tunnels of black leaves, surmounted by pinkish hills. Bushes were dotted with white petals that smelled of jasmine so fresh I could have bottled it. I helped my mother open the bottle of wine and poured her a glass. She basked in the moment, entranced with the sun, closing her eyes and angling her face toward the light. For a woman whose strong suit wasn't patience, my mother never failed to notice a good moment when she had one. After a sip of wine, she could talk about the things she tried to avoid. "He would have ruined your whole life," she said, apropos of nothing.

"Noah?" I asked, taking fork and knife to a grilled onion in aluminum foil.

"He was on the wrong path. I just felt so sorry for you," Mom said, swirling the wine in her glass. "You faced an awful choice with that pregnancy. Damned if you did, damned if you didn't."

"Then why won't you talk to me about it?"

"I have been."

"How so?" In twelve days, she'd hardly spoken the word "abortion."

My mother tipped her Ray Bans and looked up at me with pale green eyes. "Well yeah, Kass! I told you to finish the business with Will-B, remember?"

I coughed. I tipped my water bottle upside down and chugged, but the coughing wouldn't stop. A tickle in my throat wouldn't let me speak.

"I see Will-B now and again," she told me. "Sound of your name stuns that boy alive. If I'm not mistaken, I believe his name is stunning you right now. You should see your smile. I don't know if I believe in soul mates, per se, but you and Will-B—"

"Mama, please."

She shook her head and lifted her eyebrows as if to say, *I don't know what to do with you.*

"Unfinished business, honey." The wine had loosened her up. "Sit down and have a direct adult conversation with him. You're an alpha dog, so be an alpha dog. Tell him you love him. This shouldn't be difficult."

Will-B's email was still sitting in my inbox, unattended. Before bed, I had reread my favorite sentence on my cell phone: *I often find that you are in my thoughts which is kind've [sic] weird because we haven't really seen each other much of [sic] the past decade.* The correspondence I had hoped for—that he thought of me maybe a quarter as much as I did of him—had arrived at precisely the wrong time. My mind had been

free of suspicious thoughts for three weeks, ever since my forgiveness exercise at Rachel's Vineyard. Finishing the business couldn't
involve an exchange that remotely resembled cheating, not even a
flirty email, or else I'd relapse into lunacy, checking Greg's receipts
and monitoring him for unfamiliar mannerisms.

"I can't finish any business, Mom. I'm with Greg."

"Greg is wonderful, but he's not for you—although he's got a little
bit of Will-B in him." She pinched pointer and thumb in the universal
sign for "small." "He's charming, has a sweet smile, and adores you.
But he's not career-oriented and he doesn't dance. You can't marry a
man who doesn't dance. Your dad's a complicated person, but he sure
could dance. And there's no better dancer than my husband."

"If we may shift the subject just slightly"—away from her two marriages and my failed romance and onto a lighter note—"may I ask
what's keeping you from talking to me about my actual abortion?"

"I don't know," she said, studying some point in the distance. "I
didn't talk to my mother about half the things you talk to me about
today. Back then, you just lied to keep them happy. And they lied so
the neighborhood wouldn't talk." She hearkened back to the day my
father slipped an engagement ring on her finger—"My mother takes
me by the hand and parades me around the country club, diamond
first, bragging to everyone that I'm a virgin! Your dad and I lived together! Nana knew that."

"Wait. You *lived together*?" I asked, shocked. I filled her wine glass
again. All the way to the rim. "I assumed you were a virgin bride and
I had to be an innocent flower like you. I go up north to college only
to find out that the girls there had been doing it for years."

"Well, anyway," Mom said, drawing out the word *w-e-l-l-l-l-l-l* and
arching her neck back to tan herself. (It was 7 P.M.) *Well, anyway* was
her go-to transition. It meant: conversation over. *Well, anyway* had
many uses: to maneuver out of difficult talks, to avoid an awkward

beat, to stop sadness. My girlfriends had told me that their mothers of the Move-On Generation—the same generation from which a certain militant strand of feminism had emerged—had their own such phrases: "Keep moving." "Forward march." "What's done is done."

"You think that's why Betty Lee told Granddad that we were out here in California researching fertility rituals?" I asked. When my mother's father, a Southern Baptist Republican, started calling the family to investigate the catalyst for our road trip, Betty Lee—my mother's cousin—had concocted a fib that I was researching rituals to improve fertility in the United States.

"I talked to Betty Lee about that screwy rumor," she said, with a groan. "She's got an abortion blind spot. I told her, it can happen to anybody." She took another swig. "I just think you're kind of amazing."

"You do?" The wine must have been talking.

"Don't be silly," she said, slapping my leg.

I wanted to get a tattoo on my face that said KIND OF AMAZING. I wanted to frame a sign on my office wall that said KIND OF AMAZING. I wanted to run around the vineyard yelling, MY MOM THINKS I'M KIND OF AMAZING. I welled with gratitude for our partially satisfying, slightly mystifying mother-daughter conversation about virginity myths and accidental pregnancy.

"How did it happen, exactly, with Noah?"

"Do you really want to know?"

"No," she said sharply, shaking her head. She polished off her wine, still clutching the glass with both hands, and became serious again.

"Kass," she said, "tell me the truth. Do you blame me for not preparing you to not get pregnant?"

Did I? Surprisingly, embarrassingly, the answer was yes. A little yes. It wasn't like I sat up at night, thinking, *If only my mother had spiked my water supply with birth control or given me a crash course in sex ed while fortifying me with the feminine divine before college, all would have been well.* I hadn't even noticed that I blamed her until she asked me directly. She had reached inside my head, plucked the blame out like a stubborn splinter, and held it up in front of me. And now the blame vanished. Because I'd had all the information I needed to prevent my pregnancy. Even when I was nineteen and sitting at the health clinic, getting turned down for an IUD, I knew I should have demanded it from the reluctant consultant. A voice inside of me had said: the professional is wrong, condoms won't work. It said: you need this birth control now. I ignored the voice.

In some ways, that moment in the health clinic cut me deeper than the abortion itself. It cut into the wire on my tin can phone line to God: my intuition. And every single time I denied a feeling that something wasn't right, or that something was right, I degraded my self-esteem, I copped resentments, I destroyed happiness. Every single time. I felt angry when it turned out that my intuition was correct and I had ignored it. Naturally, I projected my guilt onto the easiest person to blame: my mother.

It was wild, all the messages that train women that our gut feelings are wrong, and how easily I fell prey to the idea that someone else, some expert, some older person, some person I gave authority, knew what I needed more than I did. Every damn day, it's a practice to get down with God in my gut. I could trust my underground voice.

"No, Mama," I said. "I don't blame you."

(As of three seconds ago.)

Telling my mother face-to-face that I didn't blame her for my pregnancy made a layer of tension fall from my body. It felt like removing a heavy coat.

"A mother wonders," Mom said, wrapping one arm around my goose-bumped shoulder as we sat at the weathered picnic table, surrounded by vineyards, the sun dropping behind us.

- 13 -

ANIMAL THERAPY

SIX YEARS AND FIVE MONTHS AFTERWARD — Greg and I adopted a dog that fall. We sat side-by-side on our black love seat, browsing canine headshots on my laptop. I searched for gentle giants, big enough for my big emotions: mastiffs, Newfoundlands, Saint Bernards. Much to my surprise, Greg preferred small dogs.

"How about him?" I pointed at a mastiff with a wrinkly grandpa muzzle. The absurd size of our graduate housing apartment, huge for Manhattan, could easily accommodate the two-hundred-pound dog on the screen. After all, the tenant above us had a white Great Pyrenees that she could have rented out for pony rides.

"Nah," said Greg, emphasizing his preference for small dogs. "How 'bout him?" He pointed at a twenty-pound beagle with a condition called "dwarfism." Black fur with legs like long white flapper gloves.

"I'm in love." I fell in love with all dogs.

Next thing I knew, we had a dog. Our twenty-pound "grief companion," estimated to be six years old, had ridden in the front seat of a pickup truck from Ohio to our living room, furnished with street junk. Sopping wet from a bath, he was zipping around our apartment like a tuna fish, jumping up on the black love seat and then taking off down the hall, his toenails tapping the hardwood floors.

"What should we call him?" asked Greg, chasing our slippery critter with an open green towel. "Gaw," he said, before I could answer. "It's like trying to catch a bug."

"Bug," I said, sipping a cup of coffee, "is his name."

Greg arranged a fluffy plaid doggy mattress next to his side of the bed while I took two soup bowls down from the cupboard and put them in the hallway, filling one with water and the other with dog food. The first night, Bug climbed into our bed, poking his furry head out of the covers, right between us.

I'd jumped right back into the busyness of everyday life: Facebook feeds, trips to the grocery store, plus the graduate school grind of teaching undergraduates and reading hundreds of assigned pages— all up in my head again. Much to my chagrin, grief would not happen to me "accidently" any more than I'd "accidentally" get rock hard abs. Regular exercise, no fewer than thirty seconds a day as Ava had instructed, was the workout plan.

Bug would be my li'l helper.

The second night, Greg went off to work the overnight shift at the television station. I had Bug alone, just like I wanted him. I was standing in the bedroom, looking down at the panting Bug, his black coal lump eyes searing into me.

"Bug," I said. "I am experiencing deep sadness."

He just blinked at me with his little square head, his red tongue hanging out.

"Do you understand me?"

He glanced around the room, even rubbernecking behind him, like, *Is everyone else seeing what I'm seeing?* I was seeking that cinematic moment when nobody but your dog understands your sorrow. Sensing your sorrow, he snuggles up to you and lays his head on your shoulder, as if to say, *There, there buddy.*

I sat cross-legged on my bed and set my timer for thirty seconds anyway, expecting Bug's intuitive canine senses to pick up the signal about a certain girl who needed a certain friend. I closed my eyes and prayed for anyone who might think I was being melodramatic, including me. Because part of me didn't want to finish grieving. The tiny destroyer of love inside of me wanted to hold my choice against me in bleak years to come. As long as I resisted grief, she twisted any dark day back to my nixed motherhood and said, "See? You should have had that baby."

She had to go. Grief would tap her magic wand and make her disappear.

The timer buzzed. Nothing had happened. I went to wash my face, feeling unsuccessful. When I came out of the bathroom dabbing my face with a towel, Bug had stretched his small body across both pillows on the bed, front paws all the way on the left side and back all the way on the right side, so that there was nowhere to lay my head. "Come on, Buggy," I said, patting my legs, prompting him to scoot over. He didn't budge. I started to lift him up, putting one arm over his back and the other under his chest. He curled up his lips, bared his teeth, and bit me on the hand. I jerked away and screamed. Bug tumbled down to the bed, landing on all fours and returning to his pillows. Ugh. I stretched out with my bare feet hanging off the side, crying out of frustration, with dots of blood on my hand.

What ever happened to *there, there, buddy?*

I sat again the next morning for half a minute, trying not to intellectualize the loss and the terror I felt about the life I had stopped. So began my practice of sitting for thirty seconds a day, not thinking, not meditating, not doing shit else besides waiting for heartache to move through me.

In a used bookstore with a high ceiling crammed with musty-smelling paperbacks, I tugged out a copy of C. S. Lewis's book *A Grief Observed* and opened it and read the first two lines: "No one ever told me that grief felt so like fear. I am not afraid, but the sensation is like being afraid."

Grief felt like an extended period of disorientation, like being lost. The thing about grief is that it is not a narrative. I project stories and meaning onto everything I see, but grieving required stopping this entirely and being in the mysterious alchemy of grief, which was terribly uncomfortable. I had no context for the life I was moving toward. Progress. I walked and walked, aimlessly, Bug tugging on the leash. I found grief to be less about "doing" and more about being vigilant about my sneaky brain's tendency toward denial and circumvention. Bingeing on four seasons of *Gossip Girl,* for instance. And all five seasons of the television show *Friday Night Lights.* I developed a borderline deranged crush on Taylor Kitsch, who played Tim Riggins, the alcoholic teenage football star with mommy issues that made my friends uncomfortable. Grief would wait.

On the floor of the living room, I breathed in the dark and held onto nothing, no representation of loss. I listened. I listened to feet shuffling through the hallway outside my door; the elevator's ding-ding; the new mother next door whose colicky daughter screamed in concert with an elderly person in the building behind my apartment. Bug came and snuggled up next to me so that his body was parallel to mine. Faces came to me: my grandmothers, my dead friends. Places, too, like the Strawberry Lane house. I breathed waves up to my head. I breathed the love pulsing through the city, the other New Yorkers who might be lying in the dark, listening to grief, too. This lasted off and on for about five months. Then, abruptly, on an ordinary morning, it was over. The gray film over my brain had dissolved.

A curious thing happened when I finished grieving: Greg and I had stopped having sex.

I had started planning my wedding to Greg pretty early in the relationship, say probably one or two hours after he told me he wasn't sleeping with anyone else besides me. Now we had a dog, an apartment, furniture. And his mother referred to me as her daughter-in-law. Greg never made me feel trapped; he gave me so much wonderful magical space that I could disappear in the library for hours on end, eat dinner with my guy friends, do anything besides date other people.

I blamed the sex drought on my thirty seconds of grief and our mismatched schedules. Come to think of it, I couldn't remember the last time we'd done it. I brought my concerns to Greg's attention, suggesting that we let Bug sleep on the floor instead of snuggling between us in bed a couple nights a week. He disagreed. I lit sexy aromatherapy candles. I smudged our sheets with a sage wand. I bought lacy underwear, had Brazilian waxes, suggested we play a self-explanatory game I called "Sex for Thirty Nights." Greg declined.

After many months of this sort of effort, we rented a Woodstock cabin with friends of ours—a married couple. That night, after Greg gently rebuffed my advances, I turned my back to him and Bug, tucking my hands under the pillow, listening to the headboard banging against the wall in the next room. By some miracle, I didn't take it personally or feel like something was wrong with me because my boyfriend would rather have our dog sleep between us than have sex with me. But I didn't stop wanting to have sex.

- 14 -

MANIFESTO OF THE THREE BILLION SLUTS

One million women in France have an abortion every year.

Condemned to secrecy, they have them in dangerous conditions when this procedure, performed under medical supervision, is one of the simplest.

These women are veiled in silence.

I declare that I am one of them. I have had an abortion.

—SIMONE DE BEAUVOIR, "MANIFESTO OF THE 343 SLUTS," APRIL 5, 1971

SEVEN YEARS AFTERWARD—I watched the letters march across the computer screen as I typed an imaginary email that I hoped to receive: "Dear Kassi Underwood, Your essay will be published in the *New York Times* on July 28th. Signed, The Editor." With Bug curled up under my desk, his warm chest expanding on my feet, I printed out this egomaniacal missive and cut it out with a pair of flimsy kid scissors, turning it into a slip of paper an inch in width, and taped it to the top edge of my laptop.

One year after breakfast with the Baker Babe, I began to write my story. The "Modern Love" column in the *Times* had more than one million readers. Why, a sane person might ask, would I want to publish an article about my abortion for a million strangers to read? Because it was the story I wanted to read, one that would implicitly say: It's okay to suffer and it's okay not to suffer. It's okay to define what suffering means to you and it's okay if it's indescribable. It's okay to talk about your pregnancy without talking about your abortion. It's okay if your ambitious longings turned out to be anticlimactic. It's also okay to Facebook-stalk your ex in a crazed obsession with his newborn daughter. It's okay to search for some ineffable thing that might make you feel better and not to find it in the obvious places.

In 1971, Simone de Beauvoir and 342 French women signed a document declaring that they had obtained illegal abortions. It was called "Manifesto of the 343," colloquially known as the "Manifesto of the 343 Sluts." Across the world, humans have had approximately three billion recorded abortions in the past fifty-five years alone. Literally *billions* of living people shared in this experience together. Three Billion stood for all of us. And I wanted a manifesto for all of us.

The majority of my girlfriends in New York, maybe 70 percent, had casually mentioned having terminated a pregnancy, but I'd never had the guts to ask them to chronicle the tale. *What if they don't want to tell me? What if I fall apart while listening?* But my friends were all grown-ass women and they could say no if they didn't want to talk about it. And grief itself had prepared me to listen to others' stories more fearlessly. And so what if I cried while listening?

One afternoon, after a date at the nail salon, my friend Liza and I sat together on a park bench. We wore matching rubber flip flops with tissues threaded between our toes. Liza was a writing professor with a long panel of burgundy-tinted hair. Olive-skinned and gorgeous, she wore cat eye glasses with studs at the points. Looking out over a field dotted with early spring sunbathers and children romping to and fro, we blew on our charcoal-maroon-painted fingernails and fanned our hands. I handed her six folded-up pages of my *Times* hopeful.

"What was it like when you went through it?" I asked. Liza had had two abortions. She was among my dearest friends—we'd met each other's mothers, traveled together, and worked together—and yet my mouth went dry as I asked the question.

"I was twenty-five," she told me. "I was married. I thought my husband and I would have kids maybe five years down the line. I was going to make it as a writer and have this amazing career set up before I could think about having kids. Then the doctor confirmed that I was pregnant and said, 'Well, you're married. You're at a good age. You may as well go ahead and have it.' Because I was married and a certain age, I was being talked out of terminating? I don't remember feeling any doubts, but even if I did, my decision was definitely confirmed by my then-husband, who was like, 'No.' It wasn't like we were struggling financially. He was just like, 'No.' He didn't want the responsibility. He came with me to the appointment and was on his Blackberry the whole time. He had this lets-get-this-over-with attitude. The procedure was quick and pretty painless, not anything worse than getting a tattoo."

"You're lucky," I said, blowing my nails. My abortion held the record for the worst physical pain I had yet endured.

"Yeah, it was easy for me," Liza continued. "Afterward, the nurse asked me, 'Do you want to see?'—I think she called it 'the material,' or something—and I said, 'Sure, yeah, why not?' And she said, 'We like to ask, so that way, people can see that this wasn't something that was formed.' I think they try to assuage a woman's potential guilt. Whatever word they used seemed suitable for what it was. The second abortion was after I got separated. I was twenty-seven, using a diaphragm, dating a broke poet. You remember him—"

I couldn't forget him. He destroyed her apartment after they split up, drowning in the bathtub both of her laptops, fourteen years of her journals, and the only hard copy of her forthcoming memoir.

He had also left her a voice message: "Sorry you can't come to the phone right now, seeing as your shoes are soon to be on fire." Then he torched her Accomplishment Boots, a thousand-dollar pair of platform wedges she bought to celebrate the publication of her first book. *Seeing As Your Shoes Are Soon to Be on Fire* became the title of her third book.

"He was more open than my husband. He was like, 'What if we just had a baby and tried to make it?' I contemplated it for a minute, because we were having an actual conversation. And I was like, yeah, no, it's better not to. This would be a bad decision. I didn't think about the abortions too much afterward until your project, and then I started to see more than just pro-life and pro-choice. I wondered, *What does a woman go through after abortion?* I was just relieved afterward. Did I bury feelings about it? I don't think I did. In one case, it was the wrong marriage, and in the other case, it was a relationship that was fated to end. He was drunk and terrible. I'm glad that neither of them gave me something I'm going to have the rest of my life."

Then Liza added, "I'm sure if I had the kids I would be telling a very different story right now."

"Me too," I said.

SIX WEEKS AFTER SENDING OFF MY ESSAY to the *Times,* still no word. Giving up on a publication for millions of readers, I emailed Mira Ptacin, the hostess of a literary event in Greenwich Village. I sent her my essay and asked about reading my work on the stage of the Cornelia Street Café. "Hell yes," she replied in the subject line.

When the day came, I tied a red paisley bandana around my neck and slid each arm through a faux fur vest. Greg and I shuttled downtown in a packed rush-hour subway car and then galloped down the dim-lit staircase to the basement of the café. A sultry red velvet curtain hung behind the stage. A lone microphone stood in the middle of the platform. Skinny intellectuals in thick black glasses and tweed blazers huddled around the tables, sipping tumblers of liquor and, I was sure, quoting classic Russian novels I shoulda read in elementary school. No way I was reading about my primitive postabortion melt-down in front of literary prodigies.

"I'm an idiot," I said to Greg, shaking my head, covering my face with one hand. I turned back to the staircase. "I can't do this. Let's leave."

Greg grabbed my arm, stopping me. "You have to. All your girl-friends came out to see you." He pointed across the shadowed room to a table where Liza and five more buddies were waving at me.

"But I never told them I had to go on a legit spiritual journey for healing—and it's not even over yet," I whispered. "They think I'm normal."

"I'm sure they don't think that," Greg said, with a chuckle. Point taken. A successful journalist buddy once took me to a private invitation-only bookstore haunted by living legends like writer Jona-than Franzen. In casual conversation with a young snob whose name I had yet to learn, I said, "Honey, thoughts ain't nothin' but prayers." Overhearing me, my friend grabbed me by the wrist and pulled me behind a bookcase to say, "I can't take you anywhere!"

Ten minutes after I sat down next to Liza, Mira wrapped her hand around the microphone and introduced me. Applause filled the room; my girlfriends screamed and whistled.

"I can't do it," I whispered to Greg.

"Just stand up and start walking," he whispered back, as the ap-plause faded into silence.

He took both my hands and pulled me up from my seat.

You are allowed to faint before you reach the microphone, I chanted in my head as I passed the tables of eyes. *In fact, fainting would be prefera-ble. You are allowed to stutter, stumble, fall down, and get booed.*

Onstage, I set the six sheets of paper on the podium and read the words. And I didn't faint. The audience even laughed at the jokes (and by "audience," I meant the table of my pals).

When the show was over, Mira, in a tan trench coat and red lipstick, pulled up a chair and sat next to me. "You are such a badass," she said. I thought, *me?*

She'd had an abortion herself. Over the barroom chatter, she told me how her birth control pills had failed in graduate school, early into a courtship with a dark-haired guy her mother and older sister had picked out for her on a dating website. A shotgun wedding followed. Around six months' gestation, the couple learned that their unborn daughter was suffering from a litany of irregularities and chose to terminate. She tells the unabridged version in her memoir *Poor Your Soul.* When Mira returned to school without a newborn, nobody offered condolences for the loss of her child. Meanwhile, they threw a get-well party for a student with a broken foot.

"Why her foot but not my baby?" Mira asked. Seriously.

Shortly after my café reading, I did another reading in my buddy Chloe's bohemian loft in the Hudson Valley. In the kitchen afterward, a warm brunette writer with a nose ring handed me her memoir *Some Girls: My Life in a Harem,* which contained a chapter about her abortion. "I have a feeling you'll relate," Jillian said. "Let me know what you think." A bodacious blonde memoirist in a long belted dress came into the kitchen and slung one arm around Jillian's waist. "Are we talking postabortion meltdowns?" she asked. "Because I totally had one, too."

"You, too?" I leaned forward, never so pleased to hear that someone had suffered. She reached out, grabbed my hand, and held it for a moment.

"Oh, yeah. Sobbing on the bathroom floor," she said.

On the train back to Manhattan, I sat by the window and tore through Jillian's book, dabbing my eyes with a Chipotle napkin I'd scavenged from my purse. After being a concubine for the Sultan of Brunei's brother, she moved back to Manhattan and lived with a computer nerd named Andy and adopted a python and furnished her apartment with a lopsided couch and got pregnant. In high school, she had locked arms with a group of girls to protect women from the picketers outside of clinics. She writes: "I didn't really tell Andy or anyone else how badly I wanted to keep the baby, how my heart twisted in protest against the decision my head had made." Jillian would never become pregnant again. "I suspect my abortion had something to do with the infertility, but I'm not sure. It could have been a lot of things," she wrote to me in an email. Together with her husband, she adopted two extraordinary little boys. Her second memoir is called *Everything You Ever Wanted*.

Here were the Three Billion.

While I was waiting to hear from the *Times*—and during the years to come—I became a collector of stories, creating a communal narrative from books and essays and conversations:

I'm pregnant. I just found out. I'm having an abortion on Saturday at 10 A.M., begins an essay by Jenny Kutner, whose copper IUD failed to do its job. *I guess I'm the 1 percent,* she concluded, referring to the chance of getting pregnant with an IUD in place. Her essay is titled "I'm Having an Abortion This Weekend": *I wasn't sure what to feel after I made the appointment, so I just stood still on the sidewalk for a few minutes and cried. I cried because I was overwhelmed and confused, although I wasn't at all confused about my decision.*

Injustice was written on our womb stories. Failures in birth control and sex education, lessons we should have been taught about our bodies when we were children: you can get pregnant the first time you have sex. You can get pregnant in water. You can get pregnant during your period. You can get pregnant while using a condom, especially if the condom is used incorrectly. In *Lizz Free or Die,* Roman Catholic–bred comedian Lizz Winstead recalls her high school abortion in 1979: *If I used birth control and had sex, I would be committing two sins. So I did what anyone with a shred of insight would do: minimized my sinning. I opted to commit one sin. The one that was more fun.* Renee Bracey Sherman missed a pill at the age of nineteen and heard from friends that the birth control medication remained in her body, a rumor about birth control that is not true. *I don't think the punishment for missing a pill should be to raise a kid,* she told me. *I didn't realize that if you're throwing up the Pill it's not in your system,* said Katie Stack on MTV's show "16 and Pregnant: No Easy Decision." Katie Klabusich had a low-paying job and an insurance policy that didn't cover birth control: *I chose food over birth control.*

We wrote about why we had abortions. Sometimes babies became sick before they could be born. Sometimes people simply didn't want to become parents. So many reasons resonated with mine:

—*A baby meant the destruction of everything I might become* (Molly Crabapple).

—*I was broke, unmarried, restless, with addiction problems I hadn't solved* (Susan Shapiro).

—*I had published three books by then, and none of them had sold particularly well, and I did not have the money or wherewithal to have a baby* (Anne Lamott).

—*I'm on Accutane [which can cause birth defects]. But I knew that even if I weren't on the medication, I would've made the same decision* (Toni Braxton).

—*I was afraid [that my mother] would withdraw her support for my education, send me away to avoid additional scandal, and force me to place my baby for adoption, which seemed far more brutal than abortion* (Sydna Masse).

—*We're broke kids* (Bailey).

—*I didn't have the mental capacity to deal with having a child* (Sherri Shepherd).

—*We're always the image of a black woman: we have stereotypes of welfare queens. I wanted to defy stereotypes. Also, I simply wasn't ready to be a parent* (Renee Bracey Sherman).

—*I wasn't ready. I didn't have anything to offer a child* (Nicki Minaj).

—*We'd set up our kids to fail* (Markai Durham).

—*I've been without water, I've been without lights, I've been without food. And I'm not going to put anybody else through that* (James Dramz).

—*Irregular heart structure, no brain development, and clubbed feet* (Mira Ptacin).

—*Trisomy, a triple chromosome* (Ayelet Waldman).

—*I acknowledged it as a baby and for me it was a parenting choice* (Katie Stack).

We also describe what it felt like to be pregnant:

—*Pregnancy felt like a mixture of stomach flu, clinical depression, and having a damp gray blanket wrapped around my brain* (Molly Crabapple).

—*I love milk. I drank a glass of milk and threw it up and it was still cold. I thought, This is not my body* (Renee Bracey Sherman).

—*I felt like somebody had invaded my uterus* (Katie Klabusich).

—*I raged against my body* (Mira Ptacin).

—*I felt unattractive in an entirely new way, like an honor, an important padded vessel. I loved it* (Gila Lyons).

—*I enjoyed being pregnant* (Aspen Baker).

Contrary to a common armchair theory that abortion is the sign of a doomed marriage, couples who are deeply, madly in love may very well stay deeply, madly in love. In *Bad Mother*, Ayelet Waldman writes about learning that her unborn child, whom she and her husband named "Rocketship," had a genetic abnormality. Her husband told her: *If we do what you want to do, if we have the abortion, and it turns out that Rocketship would have been healthy after all, I can live with your mistake. I can love you no matter what.* Ayelet had once notoriously confessed, *I love my husband more than I love my children*—I adored that about her. Iman Ahmed, a devout Muslim, treasured her husband's theological evaluation: *Deciding for termination, in my case, was actually the more difficult decision, or the jihad as he put it, because ending my pregnancy would mean reversing years of social conditioning.*

Sometimes the relationship isn't going to last:

—*Underneath it all, I knew Josh wasn't right for me* (Gila Lyons).
—*The father was someone I had just met, who was married, and no one I wanted a real life or baby with* (Anne Lamott).
—*He had an eighth-grade education and no job. He had already been incarcerated for drugs and was trying to make ends meet, doing the best he could* (Renee Bracey Sherman).

I loved the freedom to name the pregnancy whatever we wanted. Cells, blood, or baby. Water baby, a son or a daughter, a child, a human, a potential human, a being, an unborn. Rocketship. Guiding Light. *I began to distance myself from any maternal feelings I might have toward my unborn child* (Sydna Masse). *Although I know that others feel differently, when I chose to have the abortion, I feel I chose to end my baby's life* (Ayelet Waldman). Gila Lyons described her baby—baby is the word she uses—*as a Jewish embryo, all brain and hair.* On MTV's "16 and Pregnant: No Easy Decision," Markai Durham lectures the father of her child for calling the embryo a "thing." A single tear streams down her cheek as she gestures to her infant daughter: *A thing* can turn out just like that. Nothing but a bunch of cells can be *her.*

Religion can make an abortion sacred, or sometimes burden us with additional guilt. Gila Lyons had her procedure on a religious holiday: *A river of blood the second day of Passover. It was the best day to do it.* Iman Ahmed examines hers in the context of Muslim texts and justifies her decision by the gestational age of the fetus: *I was clearly far from the stage of ensoulment by the standards of classical Muslim jurists.* Lizz Winstead, seventeen and Catholic-educated, bargained with God: *I promise, NO MORE SEX and I will only give blow jobs.* Toni Braxton expressed, *I'd made a choice that violated every religious principle I was raised to believe.*

We chronicle the emotional afterlife—and the social expectations of our feelings:

> —*The first thing I thought when I awoke from the anesthesia was that I'd never be pregnant again, that I had just squandered my only chance at motherhood* (Lisa Selin Davis).
>
> —*I have mixed emotions right now. It hasn't been long enough for me to comprehend or understand* (Markai Durham).
>
> —*I keep waiting for my prescribed grief and guilt to come—I am braced, chest out, ready—but it never arrives* (Caitlin Moran).
>
> —*Most of my discomfort came from feeling that I should feel discomfort* (Monica Heisey).
>
> —*She shouldn't be afraid of not feeling enough because the feelings will keep coming—different ones—for years* (Leslie Jamison, calling back to her younger self).
>
> —*Because I believed abortions were a right, I pretended mine was no big deal* (Molly Crabapple).
>
> —*I wish that someone had alerted me to the harshness of the experience, acknowledged the layers of regret that built and fell away as the months and years passed* (Lisa Selin Davis).
>
> —*I would never recommend it to anyone because it comes back to haunt you* (Sharon Osbourne).

—I don't want a child. And I wouldn't be a good mother. I have no regret at all (Chelsea Handler).

Terminating a pregnancy sets off a chain of events that might not have happened otherwise:

—About motherhood, though, I was wrong. Fifteen years later, happily coupled with a wonderful man, I gave birth to my first daughter; I now have two (Lisa Selin Davis).

—What seemed tragic was that it took me until my 40s to feel together enough to bear a child. By then it was too late (Susan Shapiro).

—My abortion made me look at my life: I broke up with the boyfriend and started applying myself in school. I was granted a scholarship from Cornell University to earn my master's degree and became a writer and activist for the reproductive health of black women (Renee Bracey Sherman).

Transmen, genderqueer, nonconforming, and two-spirit people have abortions; I read one such story on the Internet: *I'm a man. And I had an abortion when I was 27* (anonymous transman).

We talk about our abortions for a zillion reasons, one of which is to find one another.

—I had an abortion when I was seventeen, and I didn't talk about it until I was thirty. I told the first person, and then she shared her own experience (Melissa Madera).

—I just want women and girls to know that you're not alone (Markai Durham).

—It saved my life to know other women who had gone through it (Ayelet Waldman).

AT THE PRECISE MOMENT MY *New York Times* essay went live on-line, I was traipsing down Main Street in my hometown, arm-in-arm with my mother and my brother, whose hundred-pound German Shepherd named Callie took long strides on her leash.

It was July 28.

I stopped on the sidewalk, pushing the screen of my iPhone with both thumbs to enlarge the microscopic words. Rusty, Mom, and Callie huddled around to look. My high school was two blocks away. I wanted to hide, but there was nowhere to go.

The story of my abortion was in the *Times.*

That night, sitting up in bed in my mother's basement, I found a lucid defense of my essay in the online comments section, under the name "Callie." (My brother also had the print edition framed.) I pored over messages from Colorado, California, Florida, Vermont, and Kentucky from women telling me about their abortions, mis-carriages, and stillbirths as well as the children they had adopted out. Hate mail came, too. "You're still a huge white trash whore from the ignorant south." And: "Too bad you didn't have a kid with your junkie boyfriend, ignorant cunt." A Christian man published a blog post on his church website saying that I'd burn in hell. But those were nothing compared to the emails from readers, mainly women, but maybe a dozen men, divulging their forbidden thoughts and emo-tions, like terror and euphoria.

Over and over, women told me the secrets that their churches called "sins." They told me about the feelings feminism forgot, the skeletons they dragged out of the bottom left corner of the broom closet and carried down Main Street in their own hometowns.

A Wall Street girl said a masseuse had been kneading her back muscles when she stopped and said, "He's waiting for you"—meaning the son she hadn't given birth to half a decade earlier. (She would later give birth to a son.) A Milton scholar with rings on every finger told me about her mother's backyard ritual to acknowledge her abortion. A bride-to-be confided in me that she hadn't told her fiancé and never would. A hardboiled German writer in baggy pants told me about an art class in which she painted three enormous circles on her canvas. The teacher asked her what the circles represented. Then she saw it: her three abortions. A journalist wore a gold hanger necklace in memory of her grandmother who had died of an illegal self-induced abortion. A quiet executive secretary wore a gold pendant necklace around her neck for her water baby.

Men told me their stories, too. A strapping Princeton-bred public school teacher told me he had a mourning meditation practice for the child he and his ex-girlfriend hadn't had in college. A bearded man in a brown sweater told me that, thirty years before, his ex-wife hadn't told him she'd been carrying his progeny until after the abortion. Not a day went by that he hadn't thought of what turned out to be his only chance to become a father. A public policy student told me about a college fling who also hid her pregnancy from him until after the termination. His mother raised him to be a feminist, but he was devastated and confused that he hadn't been able to weigh in on the decision. He was diagnosed with cancer within a year, as though his emotional anguish had metastasized. An English professor said he had knocked up a former sweetheart when he was in his twenties. No regrets for him—he just wished it had never happened. A taxi driver from Romania divulged to me that the two long rosaries hanging from his rearview mirror were in memory of his "two sons."

One morning, an email pinged my inbox from Amy, my dear sister from Rachel's Vineyard: "I saw your article in the *New York Times*," she wrote. "I wish I had the guts to say that I've felt many of the same things. That must be the true sign of healing."

15

A MARGINALLY ADVANCED UNDERSTANDING OF MY MOTHER

SEVEN YEARS, ELEVEN MONTHS, AND TWENTY-THREE DAYS AFTERWARD—"A vow of total silence, huh?" said Rosanne the groundskeeper of The Milarepa Center.

Rosanne and I had known each other for approximately thirty seconds. She welcomed me into a sunlit room furnished with long community dining tables and framed photos of the Dalai Lama in his self-tinting eyeglasses. I had come to this Buddhist hub in Vermont to meditate in a cabin for five days, alone and in silence, with one important daytrip: on Friday, which marked the eighth anniversary of my abortion, I would return to the Planned Parenthood clinic where I had had my abortion.

I needed to put my feet in the stirrups again. Just like I had eight years earlier. I needed to go back and meet my nineteen-year-old self and tell her it was okay. Because one way to heal is to return to painful scenes and inject them with love. Planned Parenthood was the closest thing I had to a grave—the clinic was sacred ground to me.

"No cell phone, no laptop, no contact with the outside world?" Rosanne continued. She had smooth skin and hair all askew, white roots blending into charcoal gray that fell over her shoulders. "Have you ever done this before?"

"No, I—" I began to cough and tried to speak again. "I—"

My entire body was buzzing like a knocked funny bone. I was also having suicidal thoughts and crying spells. I didn't mention to Rosanne that I would be withdrawing from the antidepressant Zoloft during this silent retreat in the woods. I'd started taking it five years earlier, when Noah emailed me about Jade. It had done almost nothing to improve my state of mind, but it was nearly impossible to stop taking it—I'd failed three times before because of the kick.

Still coughing, I set my grocery bag on the floor and untangled my arm from the handle of my duffel bag so I could set it down, too. I clasped my hand over my mouth and continued coughing up what felt like a tiny speck of dust. (Coughing wasn't listed as a withdrawal symptom.)

"It's an impurity," said Rosanne. "They build up over the years. Your body knows you're about to take a vow of silence. It wants to purify you. It happens."

She led me to the kitchen, pulled a cup down from a shelf, and filled it with tap water. I chugged it and wiped off my mouth.

"Your cabin's open," said Roseanne, handing me a set of keys.

The screen door clattered behind me as I hugged my paper bag of rations and head-butted a harsh Vermont wind, brutal even in April. Snow stitched down, flakes sticking to my mustard-colored ski hat, the metallic scent of winter mixing with the wild ginger of spring. I clunked across a wood plank bridge, ice edging the banks of the stream below. Then I stopped in a field and beheld my home for the next five days: an unfinished wood cabin that looked too narrow to fit a bed. A massive porch wrapped around it with plenty of room for sitting. Big blue water jug. No plumbing. Just a red outhouse about twenty yards away.

I walked up the creaking steps and let myself in. The electric heater sputtered, blowing warm air on my shoulder as I knelt down and loaded the mini-fridge with groceries, soymilk, and peanut butter. I could open both the mini-fridge and the front door while on the bed.

Scanning the tiny cabin, my silent home in the rural woods, I feared that someone would die and nobody would know how to get in touch with me. Or I would die. A bear would eat me.

You done lost your mind, I thought. *Five days. Hunkering down alone. Did you remember to bring your crack pipe?*

So I decorated. Tacked the banner of Boundless Love and Boundless Light from the *mizuko kuyo* ritual to the wall. Set the bottle of Living Water from the naming ceremony on the sill. Fished my running shoes out of my bag and dropped them by the door. A small town was at the bottom of the gravel hill—I'd jog, see some humans, and shoot endorphins into my brain.

Once the room was arranged, I ceremoniously lit a candle on the windowsill and took a risk I had never taken before, according to my family: the risk of silence. For the next ninety hours, I would not speak. (With two important exceptions . . .)

Not quite sure what to do with myself, I stood at the front door, watching a bird with a power tool beak peck at a tree. "Wow," I said out loud. "What kind of bird is that? Shit! Dammit." Nature was too stimulating. So I tucked myself under the covers with a spoon and an open jar of peanut butter—and managed nearly six minutes of silence. Then: "This is really good peanut butter."

Night fell within the hour.

I had to pee, and the outhouse was dark and there was snow on the ground and there were bears. It was 7 P.M. I held it and pulled the covers up to my neck, crying with loneliness. *What was I doing here?* Why had I come to the woods of Vermont to spend five days alone while withdrawing from Zoloft—just so that I could go back to the clinic?

What was the meaning of my silent retreat in the woods? I didn't know. But I did know. I was still trying to force myself to come up with a verdict about my abortion, as if I had to be "decided" about whether I had made the right decision at the end of my pilgrimage. As if I would emerge from the woods with an answer to the question to which Jesus basically said "no comment," the Qur'an bypassed, and rabbis had debated for millennia: was abortion right or wrong?

I had no answer. What I had now was a God who made himself annoyingly apparent to me in specific situations. I mean, this guy was so obvious that I couldn't get him to stop giving me input—never about other people's lives (that wouldn't be God—that would be ego, unless someone asked me directly), but about what to do in each moment, the action or nonaction that would give me the utmost peace, even if the directions seemed like tall orders. The answers hit my solar plexus, the spot between my boobs and my womb. They were clear, direct, and always possible. There wasn't a verdict about my termination because the decision was over. Instructions applied to what could be done in this moment. It was like God was saying, *There is nothing to decide.*

I pondered all sorts of things in the dark—it was only 7:20 P.M., for Chrissake. In particular, I thought about the fate of my relationship with Greg. All I could think was how much I loved him, and how grieving strengthens you to let go of the ones you love when it's time to let go.

The next morning, I rose with the sun and pulled wool socks on my feet and a hat on my head and then went outside on my side porch, which was wider than the cabin itself. I turned on the Coleman stove. The antidepressant withdrawal symptoms shocked my brain as I boiled water for tea, poured it into a mug, and went back inside to begin my final assignment for Rabbi Rayzel Raphael.

Over the course of the past two years, we had exchanged exactly

120 emails, most of them containing her instructions for spiritual exercises. I would make a mental note of her directions and then run over to the navy blue meditation cushion to do the exercises she assigned, and then run back to the computer and dispatch an update, await her single-phrase reply, and then run back to do another exercise any time the first try didn't "take." That "not taking" happened a lot.

Her favorite exercise was "automatic writing." Automatic writing is believed to have been the method used to pen the Zohar, the foundational text of mystical Judaism, or Kabbalah, a tradition that has garnered followers such as Madonna, Britney Spears, and Demi Moore. The Zohar expands upon the Torah so that its readers can transcend the trap of knowledge and experience enlightenment.

Automatic writing is fairly simple: You take out a pen and paper. Using your dominant hand, you jot down a question. Then you pass the writing utensil to the opposite hand, and wait for your hand to write the answer. Make no effort, as your hand will "automatically" transcribe the reply.

Rabbi Rayzel speculated that the answer would come sometimes from God, sometimes from the higher self, sometimes from the soul of the baby. I'd sit on my meditation cushion in my office overlooking the airshaft with a notebook in my lap and light a tea candle on the windowsill. Then I'd ceremoniously begin scribbling with my non-dominant hand, expecting extraordinary answers to emerge. My answers came out looking like a ransom note written by a five-year-old.

Rabbi Rayzel suggested that a cabin in the Northeast Kingdom of Vermont might be more conducive to her exercises than an apartment in Manhattan that shares a wall with a fire station. She bid me to ask three more important questions on my sojourn into the woods. She would hold off meeting me for the final ritual she had planned for me until I had received a satisfactory response. Unlike every other expert I consulted, Rabbi Rayzel was priming me for a celebration.

I sat on the floor of the cabin and opened my notebook and wrote my questions. Then I took the pen in my left hand, which "automatically" wrote the answers in all caps.

> *Is there something you need in order to move on?*
>   A PROPER BURIAL
> *Is there something I need in order to move on?*
>   [ILLEGIBLE.]
> *Where do I need to open to love in my life?*
>   YOUR MOTHER.

I BROKE MY NINETY HOURS OF silence by calling a "good Catholic psychic medium" in Illinois before my drive to Planned Parenthood. I'd never called a psychic before, but what would a journey of healing after abortion be without an attempt to communicate with the dead?

I didn't tell the psychic why I was calling. She asked me whether I was a mother. I hesitated. Then she said, in a monotone with a blunt midwestern accent, "Christ has the baby and it was a little girl. This was supposed to happen. You had to birth that baby into uteral form, not physical form, so that the soul could expand in knowledge. And you needed to make this connection with her so that you could learn lessons."

The psychic told me that the girl projected herself as seven years old, which would have been right if everything had aligned. "She was your mother in a past life, and she gave you up for adoption. You wanted to know what it was like to be a mother without having a child." Then she said, "Did you have a girl's name picked out? Did you think of varying the name at some point?"

"Yes," I replied.

"She does not like the new name."

"Judah?"

"Yeah, not Judah. Add an L. She's suggesting Jadel."

The name Jadel means "one who is punctual": one who arrives at the agreed-upon or proper time.

I asked whether "Jadel" forgave me.

"No," the psychic replied. "She's telling me there's nothing to forgive."

"Thank you." Until I heard that there was nothing to forgive, I hadn't let myself know that I'd been afraid of not being forgiven.

"She knows where her place is, and that's heaven. She will watch over your children when you have them."

I STARED OUT THE WINDSHIELD OF my car at the chain-link fence behind the clinic. The wires of the fence were encased with rust and overgrown with weeds. I remembered a row of neatly pruned bushes the color of emerald. I remembered Noah sitting next to me in this parking spot, eight years earlier, his grabbing my clammy hand from the passenger's seat and kissing it.

"Are you ready?" he asked me.

I had wanted so badly to know how I'd feel when it was over, but the only person who could answer that question was my future self.

Here I was.

A security system had been installed. The receptionist typed and answered phones behind bulletproof glass.

"Hi," I said through a round black speaker. "I was a patient here once."

"Come on in," she said, pressing a buzzer. She wore scrubs and wire frame glasses on a button nose. She didn't seem surprised to see a former patient stopping by.

"I had an abortion here eight years ago, today."

I gave her my name. The receptionist tapped on her computer.

"Wow, yep. Eight years ago today. You want your records?"

"Please," I said.

While she worked on the records, a nurse led me to the room where I had had an abortion. She told me to take as long as I needed and shut the door behind her. The room was more spacious than I remembered. I climbed on the exam table, the paper crinkling as I got situated, and stuck the heels of my green boots in the stirrups. I lay back and looked at the ceiling.

I was underwhelmed. How simple the appointment had been. How much of my experience had to do with my afterlife, my interpretation. I wondered how different it would have been had I found a memoir in the library, had I told the priest in church when I was pregnant, had I known how many of us carry this story with us. I wanted to say some socially inappropriate but perfectly reasonable shit after my abortion. I wanted to be able to say that I'd been pregnant, and tell people, and have them ask me about those eight weeks while a liquid gold tide surged up in my heart. I didn't realize it until now, but I had wanted to talk about the pregnancy—this spark of life inside of me that reminded me that I was born with that spark. The word "abortion" made it sound like the only meaningful thing about carrying the spark was that it had ended. But the world's not set up for me to casually drop over dinner that I was pregnant temporarily without inviting another uncomfortable conversation.

I gave life for eight weeks. Eight years later, I was back at the last place where I gave birth.

Maybe earth isn't the only place where there's life. Maybe this world isn't our home. Maybe this world isn't the only world we've got. Maybe my body isn't the most important thing about me.

It was an eight-week assignment. And now I had an experience with mother love.

Here's how I understand mother love: taking on the burden of judgment and shame and isolation and ostracism and mental torture and physical torture to spare a child from pain. People might not understand why I do what I do. They don't have to.

My records came in an envelope that I tore open with a fingernail. It wasn't twins. It was a single pregnancy, two months along. A girl.

BUNDLED UP IN A BLANKET, I sat on the front porch of the cabin clutching a warm mug of tea with both hands and asked for a sign that I was ready for the last ritual with Rabbi Rayzel. It was still Friday, my last night before I'd head back to New York.

Towering green pines overlaid the white sky. The air froze to my skin. I suited up in my sneakers and headed out on a run through the Main Street of Barnet, Vermont: population 1,708. The church sign read BACK IN JUNE.

One business stood out: a bold purple shop called Samadhi Cushions, with a storefront of braided red columns. A hanging sign out front read "Est. 1975."

Who shops there? I wondered on my first jog up the hill.

Seriously, who keeps this store alive? I wondered on the next trip.

On my last run, I thought, very forcefully this time, *WHO SHOPS THERE?*

Then I remembered: *I shopped there.*

The Year I Began Meditating, I had ordered my navy blue meditation cushion online from Samadhi Cushions. I had been sitting on my cushion for five years, and although it was now lumpy and stained with coffee spills, it was a comfort. Whether I was making an offering to Jizo, making nice with clinic picketers at Rachel's Vineyard, or making progress with my mother in California, I always had the cushion to return to. Now, by pure coincidence, I had circled back to its extremely rural origin.

As far as signs go, it couldn't get more obvious than an actual sign—one that symbolized completion to me.

But I did get a more obvious sign.

The next morning, I opened the door to a crisp blue April day, all ready to go, carrying bags in my arms. Just before I switched off the light, I backed up and read a laminated strip of yellow paper that must have been mounted above the door of the cabin all week: *It is said in the Ksitigarbha Dasacakra Sutra that whoever sees, hears, remembers, or touches this mantra will be purified of all negativity and gain freedom from rebirth in the lower realms.*

I Googled "Ksitigarbha." The bodhisattva who guides aborted beings to the light—known in Japan as Jizo.

MY MOTHER SAT LIKE A QUEEN on my love seat in tall black boots with Bug curled up in her lap. I had a white envelope in mine.

"I have something to tell you," I told her.

"Dear God, what is it?"

"Well, you aren't aware of this, but when I was in college, I used the money you sent me for fixing my car to pay for my abortion. I was wrong to use your money to end my pregnancy without telling you, and I'm sorry."

Her face collapsed. She thumped one hand over her heart. "Kassi! Don't scare me like that," she exclaimed. "I thought it was something *bad.*"

Ha—I loved her.

"I owe you $400," I continued.

"You owe me a lot more than that," she said, with a frisky smirk.

I handed her the envelope full of cash, a portion of my tax return that year, but she put both hands in the air as if prompted by a police officer and said, "Put that away!"

"Come on, Ma. I had a revelation and now I'm paying you back. It's symbolic."

"It can be symbolic of you going and buying a nice dinner for yourself."

"I don't drink. I don't eat animals. I couldn't find a four-hundred-dollar dinner if I wanted to. How about I take you out for a nice dinner?"

"No, no. I got it—" She wagged her finger at me, clearly proud of her next proposition. "Use that money to fly yourself home to Kentucky."

"Okay."

"Come on home," she said, "and finish the business with Will-B."

16

WILD WOMAN

EIGHT YEARS AND TWO MONTHS AFTERWARD — Before I finished the business with Will-B, I had one the last ritual to do. But Rabbi Rayzel politely refused to schedule said ritual until I had interpreted my "automatic writing" exercises. So I walked around my lamp-lit apartment, squinting at my spiral notebook, trying to read the illegible black squiggles that were supposed to answer the most pressing question: What did I need in order to move on?

I set the notebook upright on the kitchen table and tried to read it from the other side of the room. Then I held the page tightly from end to end. I looked at it upside down and right side up. What *did* I need to move on? Finally, I saw it.

The word was SOCKS.

"SOCKS?" I said out loud. "Why would I need SOCKS?"

A euphemism for condoms? Nay, the message had to be more germane than that. At 1:02 A.M., I emailed the answers to Rabbi Rayzel and told her I had no idea why I would need "socks" when I had a whole drawer full of them. Right after I hit "send," a clue came to mind: While I was on the exam table, moments before my abortion, I had asked the nurse to take off my socks.

And yet, my socks epiphany didn't tell me why socks would help me move on—I emailed Rabbi Rayzel to report the mysterious coincidence in case she had insights. Then she wrote back: "You need to put your socks back on."

Rabbi Rayzel told me that when we had first met over the phone and I had told her about my predicament, she had pictured my two feet running in opposite directions. The old socks symbolized the old path. Thinking conflicting thoughts. I had lost my way. Getting lost had nothing to do with the precise choice that I had made—it was the fact that I had to make it in the first place, with no preparation, no education in choice. But I don't believe in decisions anymore. I believe my gut tells me exactly what to do and sometimes I pretend not to hear it or I find its instructions hard to believe. When I was pregnant, I was afraid. I was afraid of making the wrong choice. I was afraid of being an outcast. I was afraid to do what I knew I must do. Maybe the only real choice is whether I'm going to listen to my gut.

Losing my mind was the only way for me to see how my mind had commanded me to walk in useless directions. Now it was time to put my socks back on.

Rabbi Rayzel emailed me a second assignment to prepare for the ritual: "You need a new code for living. A new constitution."

What, I had to know, did a personal constitution have to do with old socks?

I found out what when I opened *Abortion and Judaism*. It was an emerald green paperback by Rabbi Daniel Schiff. Schiff told me (because books talk to me) that Jewish law—the constitution of Judaism—is known as halakhah. This freaked me out: The word halakhah means to go, to walk. The halakhah says how a person should walk through the world. How did the little writer in my pen know that a new pair of SOCKS would be the perfect symbol for walking through the world with my new personal constitution?

I turned the page in Rabbi Schiff's book: I wanted to know about the laws on abortion in Judaism. Judaism doesn't have a finalized set of rules—the halakhah has a collection of debates among rabbis who lived in different centuries and added their own insights to the Torah. Over two thousand years, various rabbis interpreted and reinterpreted scripture about abortion without reaching a consensus. Each situation calls for a specific interpretation. Schiff writes: "A competent rabbinic authority must be consulted in order to determine the halakhic answer to any real-life abortion question."

Rabbi Rayzel summoned fifty "Wild Women" from her Rosh Hodesh group. "Women Needed for a Ritual About Abortion—Confidential," was the subject line of her email. She called on them to gather together as witnesses, which would give our ritual "more punch," as she put it. Responses poured in from Hebrew priestesses and rabbis with names like Wing and Hawk. Some emailed me with their own stories; others sent encouragements.

Four women would travel to Rabbi Rayzel's house to be witness.

I wanted to understand how Jewish abortion rituals came to be. In 1973—a watershed year for women—a feminist named Arlene Agus set out to find Talmudic evidence of the role of women in Judaism. She unearthed a connection between women and Rosh Hodesh, the Jewish festival of the new moon. Eager to spread the word, she penned an article that would ignite an international phenomenon to celebrate femininity: "This Month Is for You." Jewish women began gathering all over the planet when the moon turned dark. Over heaping feasts, they chatted about spiritual practice, careers, parenting, marriage, womanhood, G!d, love, and sex.

Before 1973, Jewish rituals honoring feminine transitions had been nonexistent, but a citation in the Talmud provided undeniable evidence of a woman's right to this holiday, a right that "predates feminism," as Agus put it. Not only did they chat, but Rosh Hodesh groups also presided over rituals to honor childbirth, miscarriage, divorce, and menopause. These new rites held legitimate religious meaning because women studied the Talmud and the Torah with flexible interpretations of the texts, drawing upon spiritual matriarchs from the Bible and elemental symbols like fire, earth, and ice.

In 1983, Rabbi Rayzel joined her first Rosh Hodesh group in Jerusalem. Thirty years old and single, she sat at a kitchen table with a group of women, their legs tucked neatly beneath the chairs. They sipped tea and ate kugel, a kosher casserole. It was there with her Rosh Hodesh group that Rayzel planned her very first ritual. The name "Rayzel" finds its origins in the name Rachel, the spiritual matriarch of the Jewish people, who died during childbirth. Rachel offers hope to women wishing to conceive because she had to try so hard to have two children. Her husband, Jacob, buried her body between Jerusalem and Bethlehem. Her tomb is revered as the third most holy site in Judaism.

Rayzel and a friend from the Rosh Hodesh group found a spool of the strings used to make tzitzit—the tassels attached to the corners of a traditional Jewish man's garment—and dyed the strings red. Then they took a pilgrimage to Rachel's tomb, where Rayzel wound the strings around the tomb seven times, praying that she would become a mother. Rayzel suddenly felt electrified with the presence of Shekhinah, the feminine aspect of G!d.

Inspired by the power of ritual, Rayzel would be ordained and be transformed into a rabbi of many trades—a painter, counselor, teacher, singer-songwriter, silk shawl designer, children's book author, and oracle-card designer. But only within the previous eleven years had women been ordained as rabbis. (With one exception—a pioneering badass in Germany in 1935.) The first female Reform rabbi was ordained in 1972. The first female Reconstructionist rabbi was ordained in 1974 (this is the movement in Judaism that Rayzel associates with). Conservative Judaism ordained the first female rabbi in 1985. Orthodox Judaism does not ordain female rabbis to this day.

So when the rabbinate entered Rayzel's mind, it was a slightly revolutionary thought. And it was while she was in rabbinical school that she designed the first recorded abortion ritual.

WHEN I CONGRATULATED RAYZEL ON PENNING the first Jewish abortion ritual in 1992, she immediately emailed a mass of feminist rabbis, asking whether anyone had recorded a ritual before that year. No one had. After Rayzel, the next recorded ritual appears in 1998, developed by Rabbi Amy Eilberg. Serving as a hospital chaplain, she began to meet women who had terminated pregnancies and created a ritual for them. It was published in *The Rabbi's Manual* of the Rabbinical Assembly.

In 2000, a British rabbi named Sylvia Rothschild published a three-part ritual that begins before the abortion. In *Taking Up the Timbrel: The Challenge of Creating Ritual for Jewish Women Today,* she includes a meditation for a woman to read directly after she makes the decision, while she is still pregnant. It begins with these words: "When David fled from his pursuer, he knew that there was but a step between himself and death. He asked, 'What have I done? What is my iniquity that I am now forced to make this choice?' And he was reassured; there was no sin."

Next she offers a prayer, which includes the following words: "I ask you God to hear me, to judge me favorably, to respond to my pain and distress. Have compassion because of Your own greatness, and because of our ancestors who trusted in You. Give me wholeness of heart so that I will love and revere you, and then I shall never lose my self-respect, nor be put to shame, for you are the power that works to save me."

Throughout the seven days following an abortion, Rothschild suggests that the woman light a candle each day. Thirty days afterward, she suggests this prayer: "My child, my pursuer, is no more.

You, who see the unformed substance, who knows each person made in secret. Hide him under the shadow of your wings. Be gracious to us both. I cannot bring him back. One day I shall go to him, but he shall not return to me . . . . the voice of slender silence asks me, 'What am I doing here now?' David arose and comforted Bathsheba. I now comfort others and am comforted by them."

In 2004, Anita Diamant, author of *The Red Tent,* founded a full-service *mikveh* center in Newton, Massachusetts, that offers a ceremony for abortion among its roughly forty-five other immersion ceremonies. Mayyim Hayyim is bathed in light and wood like a yoga studio and has meticulously clean and kosher facilities. The baths are filled with rainwater. Before visitors submerge in the waters, they are asked to remove all clothing and jewelry (though, interestingly, acrylic nails that have been worn for more than thirty days are considered part of the body). The idea is for a woman to remove anything that separates her from the bath so that she can immerse herself completely, be cleansed and purified, and transition into the next stage of her life.

Visitors to the center browse through a notebook of ceremonies and choose one, so there is no need to reveal the specific reason for a visit, if someone has come because she has had an abortion. Mayyim Hayyim supports religious pluralism while still upholding a strict policy against Gentiles like myself bathing in their waters.

THE EVENING BEFORE THE NEW MOON, I sat facing the back of a train leaving Penn Station, with a steady rhythmic hum and several ritual objects in my big black bag. Two pairs of socks: one old, one new. And my new constitution. As the train shuttled south, I replayed a fight between Greg and me. He wanted me to move back to Austin with him as I had told him I would when he relocated for me. A black ball of sorrow expanded in my solar plexus as I stared down at my constitution and what it asked me to do. But tonight was not about my relationship. Tonight was about the thrill of being alive.

An hour later, dressed in black, down to my boots, I stepped off the platform in a quiet town outside Philadelphia, fully prepared to "move on," just like my mother wanted me to. After exchanging correspondence over two years, five months, two hundred emails, and one phone call, I finally climbed into the front seat of Rabbi Geela Rayzel Raphael's minivan. She had a firm handshake and was exceptionally laid back, with purple glasses and a stack of gold and silver earrings that curved up her ears, each in the shape of an upside down hand, symbolizing the open hand of the biblical prophet Miriam, whose power it was to stand up.

The same hands lined the ceilings in the rooms of Rayzel's house where I followed her around, loving the ruffled bellbottoms that swayed above her platform heels. We stood before a glass display case looking through our faint reflections to admire her impressive collection of goblets. I chose two for the ritual: one in the shape of a curvy goddess, and the other with "The Wilderness" inscribed on its side: "Blessed are you who brings us from the narrows into the wilderness and sustains us with endless possibilities and enables us to reach a new place." This cup would be filled with water and represent Miriam, whose piety and care for the Jews with whom she wandered through the desert inspired God to provide a moving well that nourished them on the road. When Miriam's fellow travelers were weak, she cared for them. When her fellow travelers were joyful, she taught them how to sing. The symbol of Miriam's Well—the water in the goblet—was a celebration of joy, transition, and renewal.

We bounced around the house like pinballs, back and forth in the hall, up and down the staircase, through the den and the dining room. We opened cabinets and slammed drawers and grabbed cedar incense to clear the air, crystals to represent the earth, and candles to represent fire. We built an altar in her living room, which, lo and behold, was modeled after a red tent. As Diamant imagined it in her novel, women came together in such a tent to tell stories during their menstrual cycles, when we are known to be most powerful. This ritual would be the one I had longed for at age nineteen, pale and depressed, reading *The Red Tent* on my front porch in Vermont.

Eight years later, Rabbi Rayzel led me into her kitchen. She introduced me to her husband, Dr. Simcha Raphael, a rabbinical pastor and psychotherapist who was sitting on a stool. He wore bright gold hoop earrings and a black T-shirt that read "Dads Against Daughters Dating." Their teenage daughter was wearing soccer shorts and drying dishes with a towel.

"So what did the soul tell you it needed to move on?" Rabbi Rayzel asked, casually as could be, while rummaging through a cabinet. She was referring to my automatic writing exercise in the Vermont cabin. I recited the scrawls in my notebook, verbatim. *What did the soul need?*

"A proper burial," I said, thinking, *Baby's first words.*

Rabbi Rayzel walked into a closet and then walked out, handing me a butcher knife that weighed five pounds. This was getting interesting. Together, we burst out the door and into a vast front yard with spongy grass and a circle of tree stumps over yonder. We stopped at a wall of fragrant lilies in pink and orange. Rayzel held them steady by their necks while I chopped off a bouquet's worth.

"For the grave," she said.

"Wait a minute." I broke a smile. "We're digging a real grave?" I had expected a symbolic burial, not an actual one in the ground. I didn't even know what I'd bury.

"*You're* digging a grave," she said, with a laugh. She gestured toward her wooded backyard and told me she had consecrated ground where a goldfish, frog, and hamster had already been laid to rest. "Which reminds me," Rabbi Rayzel said, "I need to find my shovel . . ."

THE GRANDFATHER CLOCK IN THE DEN chimed seven times. It was time for my ritual to begin. First, a dinner. Five Wild Women had streamed in through the various doors in the house and filed into the chairs around me. Rabbi Rayzel, Ellie, Shoshana, Nahariyah, and Jody, an energy healer. They had stories behind them and lines around their eyes in that wise crow way and voices that sagged and lifted thoughtfully. Rabbi Rayzel had prepared a magnificent feast of vegan food that covered every inch of the kitchen table: seaweed salad, avocado sushi, barbeque tofu, slaw, white bean hummus ("hhhcoo-mus"), marinated cauliflower, roasted vegetables, and rice.

They passed the dishes, hand over hand, and each told me why they had come tonight.

Rabbi Rayzel went first, eyeing me through the purple frames of her glasses while she portioned rice onto her plate with a spoon. She told me of her difficulty conceiving and how she had wound the red tzitzit strings around Rachel's tomb during the year she lived in Israel. Jewish tradition teaches that the biblical matriarch Rachel intercedes with the Holy One on behalf of women who want to get pregnant after making a pilgrimage to her tomb. When Rayzel thought she was pregnant, she went to a doctor and joyfully heard a heartbeat. But a week later, there was bleeding and the heartbeat had vanished. Undeterred, she said a simple yet potent prayer, only a sentence long: "I believe in miracles in the Holy City." And a sentence of prayer was all that her miracle required. The following week, the heartbeat returned. She had not lost the pregnancy after all. It wasn't until she gave birth that the doctor found a second placenta and understood that there had been twins: one had been lost. The other was a son she named Yigdal, who had grown to become the twenty-five-year-old man whom I had met earlier in the driveway.

While trying for a second child, Rabbi Rayzel said, she started fertility treatments and became pregnant with triplets. And suddenly, again, there were no heartbeats—and no miracle this time. She had to wait four days before having a procedure to clear the womb. "Four of the stranger days of my life," she said. "I could probably dig up the poetry. I was a living tomb." Rabbi Rayzel had created a ritual with her husband for solace after these womb deaths.

I passed her the bowl of seaweed salad, eager to hear more.

I listened closely to each woman as they shared their connections to abortion, which ran the gamut from supporting a friend in college to marching on Washington while six months pregnant. It was clear that they wanted me to know they had no judgments. Ellie, a priestess in a yarmulke with long limbs and languid movements, went last. Her teen son was in the kitchen, washing dishes with Rayzel's daughter.

"When I was with men, the few years I was with men, I never wanted to get pregnant. But then my mother passed away. And there were several more deaths in my family due to illness and suicide. After all the losses were done, I knew two things: one, that Deity existed, and two, that I wanted to become a mother." She purchased sperm from a sperm bank and inseminated herself for two years. She had three miscarriages. In one case, the baby had no heartbeat, and, like Rayzel, she had to wait several days before a procedure to clear the womb. "I grew up with show tunes. In the car, on my way to the hospital, I sang a version of "I'm Getting Married in the Morning" from *My Fair Lady*—but it went like this: *I'm getting an abortion in the morning! Ding-dong, the monitors are gonna chime!*" She laughed with compassion for her old self, recalling that she would have done anything to dissociate and lessen the pain of the loss inside of her.

What astonished me about each of these women was their affectionate and humorous self-regard. Before Ellie sang "I'm Getting an Abortion in the Morning," it hadn't occurred to me to think of disassociating from my pregnancy as an act of compassion. I just thought I'd been delusional. It seemed this was a both/and situation: honoring my humanity and that of the baby by distancing myself—in order to go through with the termination, in order to protect us both. *It's okay to be kind to yourself on the way to the clinic.* What a novel idea. Anyone having an abortion knows they will be judged all their life. They will be misunderstood and demonized. Grief and sorrow might await them. It's only decent to deal yourself a little bit of kindness en route to the clinic, something like an abortion-themed rendition of your favorite show tune.

"All those years as a straight woman, I never had an abortion, and now, as a lesbian, I do. Go figure," said Ellie. She laughed—we all laughed. Then she turned to me. "So tell us, Kassi—I know you're eating dinner, but do tell us. What's your *kavanah*?"

Noting my quizzical expression, Rabbi Rayzel explained that a *kavanah* is your intention, the direction of your heart, why you are doing something, why you are here tonight.

I told them I started off just trying not to lose my shit entirely at the age of twenty-five. Then I relayed my plan to befriend what I realized had been my seven demons: One Lost Embryo, Grief Phobia, Rage Toward Picketers at Clinics and Other Shame-Mongers, Pining After Almost-Married Ex Who's So Over It, Failure to Duplicate Mom's Story, Obsession with Motherhood and Other Goals, and Crazy Girlfriend Demon. "Once I befriended my demons, they changed. None of them ended up being what I thought they were." I told the Wild Women how I'd met with Buddhists, Christians, grief guru Ava, the Midwife for the Soul, academics, and a pro-voice peace listener and then had spent five days in the woods alone before returning to the clinic where I had my abortion.

"You went out on a quest," said Rabbi Rayzel. "You were tested and you came back a warrior. So what's your *kavanah*?"

Why was I here? Because I had quit running. Because you can run from grief and sorrow and responsibility and rush headlong into a new relationship or a new city or stalwart friends who will love you while you run, but if you want happiness, if you want love, if you want to become the figure you see in the distance, the future self calling your name, if you want to live the life you chose, one day you will have to stand still and hold all of it—scorched heart and broken brain, bones and skeletons of the past, the black wave of grief and the lucid thoughts of forgiveness. And now that I was holding all that, I wanted to know: was my abortion an act of love?

Eight years had passed since my abortion. Eight is a mystical number in Judaism. Seven marks completion, as in seven days in a week. Eight symbolizes starting over.

"It's your Hanukkah," said Ellie, referring to the eight-day celebration commemorating the dedication of the Second Temple in Jerusalem. "In this case," she added, "you would rededicate to the temple of your body."

My poor temple had been neglected for months.

We moved into the red tent that was Rabbi Rayzel's living room: the walls were painted red, the carpet was blood red, the couch was cherry red. The Hebrew priestesses gathered round and squeezed together on the couch and chairs and barstools. Rayzel and I sat in front of them on two squatty stools that reminded me of tree stumps.

"Kassi, why don't you tell us about who you were when you got pregnant."

"Okay. I was nineteen years old. A college sophomore. Reasonably competent, moral, open-minded."

"Good girl," said Rayzel.

Good girl?

"I was drinking too much, starving myself, eating pills."

"Bad girl!"

She hadn't told me that we would do a call-and-response, but now that I'd caught on, I was laughing.

"I was in the honor society, Rabbi!"

"Good girl!" She shook my hand like a kid meeting the president.

"But I drank in class."

"I would never have an abortion."

"Good girl."

"But I did."

"Bad girl. See? The abortion becomes the bad girl."

Woah. How was that idea still stuck in my head? I supposed that was what the burial was for.

I reached down and pulled out the old pair of socks from the bottom of my big black bag. Thinning at the heel, the socks were white and patterned with cherries and slot machines. The meaning of the cherries was self-explanatory. The slot machines reminded me of gambling. Terminating my pregnancy had felt like a gamble—I had no idea what would happen next, how I would feel, how I would survive if I lost my mind, so I had to take the biggest gamble of my life. Having a child would have been a gamble, too, but it wasn't the one I took.

"My grandmother, my father's mother, died a week before my first ritual. I inherited most of her clothing, including these."

I held the socks in the air like a prize fish and explained their significance.

Rayzel pointed out the symbolic value of the socks: that socks cover the soles/souls of the feet. One walks a mile in someone else's shoes. Finding your feet meant getting grounded and oriented in one's surroundings. "The old socks represent the old path. Let's bury the old path," said Rayzel, looking over her purple glasses at me.

Ellie, seated on a barstool next to me, leaned down to the ground with her long frame and reached into her bag of flutes—she had brought twenty, had sixteen more at home, all instruments a friend of hers had carved by hand—and lifted one to her lips as the group stood together and paraded out of the red tent, through the kitchen, and into the backyard, under the spell of a searing flute song.

The lawn squished underfoot as I followed the procession toward the "cemetery." We circled beneath a canopy of trees. The air smelled fresh with cut grass and mud and a hint of smoke from a barbecue.

Rabbi Rayzel, a shadow across half her face, handed me an enormous shovel with a wide silver head.

"Dig, dig, dig!" she crooned.

I balanced the tip of the shovel upon the earth and stamped my foot down on the flat part of its head. I looked up at the sky. Insects buzzed in front of the slipper moon.

"What are you leaving behind?" asked Rabbi Rayzel. "You gotta say it!"

"Shame." I pitched a shovelful of dirt behind me. It landed on the ground with a thump. I dipped the shovel back into the earth, which was both grounding and limitless.

The Wild Women chimed in. We shouted into the hole, naming the things I was burying.

"The split between the good girl and the bad girl," said Rabbi Rayzel.

"The disapproval," said Jody, the energy healer.

"INNER AND OUTER," said Ellie, Shoshana, and Nahariyah, their voices blending together.

"Confusion," said Nahariyah.

"The idea that you did something wrong," said Jody.

"Noah," I said.

"Disconnection from your body," said Ellie.

"Disconnection from your heart," said Nahariyah.

"The sense that you are alone," said Rabbi Rayzel.

"The sense that you were *ever* alone," said Jody.

As our voices settled down into the hole, the shovel rasped against a rock, making the head vibrate and my hands vibrate with it. Rabbi Rayzel passed me the pair of white socks with cherries and slot machines.

For the longest time, I couldn't decide whether I was bad or good; Lilith, the wild woman, or Eve, the domestic goddess. I remembered jogging through Austin, Texas, one afternoon, trying to burn off my depression like calories. One day, I turned left down a side road instead of going straight down Tenth Street like I usually did. In the middle of the road I came across a vulture tugging with its steely beak at the body of an albino squirrel. I stopped and studied the two of them. The sun burned a crisscross tan line onto my back. I wondered which one I was—vulture or squirrel, predator or prey, bad or good? I was both predator and prey, bad and good, one and the same.

I knelt down. The wet grass seeped through the knees of my black jeans as I placed the socks in the ground. I cupped a handful of cold, damp dirt in my hands and packed it into the grave. When the socks were completely buried, I held my hair back with one hand, leaned down, and kissed the grave three times—once for the water baby, once for nineteen-year-old me, and once for whatever came. So was my abortion an act of love? Yes. Yes, it was. I laid the lilies on top of the dirt.

I thanked my younger self—including the one from a millisecond earlier—for everything she had given me. She had suffered and toiled and taken me on this wonderful strange-ass pilgrimage. She was a f*cked-up mess, and I loved her so much. But I was going to leave that girl in the earth tonight.

"By leaving this behind," Rayzel said, "you return to the place where you are not divided, where you are centered and firm on your path. Kassi, stand in the middle of us and let us escort you to your new life."

She, the priestesses, and the energy healer sang as we filed back into the house, washing death off our hands in a glass bowl before we shunted through the door, returning to the candlelit red tent and forming a crammed circle in the flickering dark. Ellie sat on a barstool, Rabbi Rayzel and I on our stools, and Jody, Nahariyah, and Shoshana on the red couch.

"I'm getting a download," said Jody. She turned her palms up to receive the message. Her helium voice went baritone. "You owe nothing. There is nothing to forgive. Does that mean anything to you?"

"Yes," I said.

You owe nothing came to me at the Roman Catholic retreat. *There is nothing to forgive* came from the midwestern Catholic psychic.

"The first feast of the evening nourished us," Rabbi Rayzel explained, holding up a platter of food. "The second feast will give us a taste of life's complexities."

There was a hardboiled brown egg, symbolic of the mourning process and the start of a new life. Wasabi for bitterness and awareness. Beets for sweetness and the womb. Figs for fertility. Onions for strength. And chocolate for transformation.

Wasabi shocked my tongue (bitterness, awareness), followed by sugary beets (sweetness, the womb). I remembered how I used to picture myself climbing up the ladder of my bunk bed in my college dorm room, lying beside my nineteen-year-old self and holding her hand and promising her that we would be better one day—as if we were separate entities, she, a tough but lost girl who dreamed that becoming a mother and a wife would turn her into the woman she wanted to become; and me, a woman who knew better—that I could become that woman with or without children and a husband. But she and I were the same, and I imagined myself, pulling myself, through time. That was my liberation from matrimony and motherhood: not needing a husband and children, but allowing myself to want them all the same. This precious voice from the grave in the backyard was saying, "Marriage and children? That's not feminist!" But yes, it was feminist. Because being feminist doesn't mean I disavow all that's traditional and feminine. It means I've got an expanded range of possibilities.

"You got the new socks?" asked Rayzel. I presented her with my new pair of royal blue tube socks with two white stripes, dying to see how this would go. She clutched them to her face and blessed them for nearly a minute, and then passed them around the room so each Wild Woman could do the same. Finally, they returned to Rayzel's hands. She got down on one knee, while I sat on the stool above her, and began working the first sock onto my bare foot, then the second, until she had pulled both blue tube socks over my black jeans and up to my knees.

"Hear ye, hear ye," called Rayzel, standing in front of the couch. The priestesses gathered round. She beckoned me to stand on the couch in my blue tube socks. "The time has come for Kassi to declare her new constitution as a whole and unified Wild Woman."

My new constitution was not a rulebook for being "good." The quest to be good was rigged anyway. My constitution was a set of guidelines for being with God.

"The Constitution of the United State of Me," I read from a piece of paper. A constitution guides future conduct. I cleared my throat and read:

In order to form a more perfect Union, establish Justice, ensure Tranquility, provide for the Common Defense, promote the general Welfare of my heart and mind and body, and secure the Blessings of Liberty to Myself and my Posterity, I do ordain and establish this Constitution for the United State of Me.

Article I. All power herein granted shall be vested in the God within me.

Article II. Pain, loss, rejection, and suffering: these four are my friends. When they knock on my door, I invite them in and pull up a seat and feed them bowls of love and let them rest.

Article III. I hereby vow not to go around taking polls to help me make decisions, no matter how big or small. Nay, I shall sit down on my trusty meditation cushion, lob my question, and await the answer.

Article IV. My mistakes are my muses.

Article V. I shall thank my protesters—they are me in disguise.

Article VI.

Section 1. I shall grieve. I shall grieve. I shall grieve.

Section 2. Grief doesn't have a half-life or a stop time. Grief is a practice. Thirty seconds, no distractions, no analyzing.

Article VII. I shall take up some f*cking space.

Done in Convention by the Unanimous Consent of the State present the Eighteenth Day of June in the Year two thousand twelve and of the Independence of the United State of Me in my twenty-eighth year of life. In witness whereof I have hereunto subscribed one Name: Kassi.

"We'd sign that," said Rabbi Rayzel and the four Wild Women: Shoshana, Ellie, Nahariyah, and Jody.

Rabbi Rayzel stood beside me holding up the Wilderness goblet. It was filled with the water that symbolized Miriam's traveling well. "The *mikveh* waters are the Jewish sign of transformation," she said. "Miriam guarded Moses when he was put into the basket and floated down the river. She was his big sister. When the Israelites crossed the Red Sea, she was the one who sang, and she was the one who had the moving well, Miriam's Well, that nourished the tribe. So I bless you with these waters of transformation. I bless you—that you see good things, hear good things, smell good things, taste good things, and have money in your pockets."

She dipped one finger in the goblet and painted my eyelids, ears, nose, lips, and hips with cool water. "That this be the cleansing element that carries you into the world and that you interface with the world knowing that you can always come back to the well of Miriam and be nurtured in a tribe of women in time and space and song and ritual and that you are not alone and that there are many women who walk your path and that you are going to be a centerpiece for creating those sacred spaces for women to talk among themselves, who want to break their silence and shame, from out of your place of isolation, that you become a healing force to create those communities. That's the blessing."

I felt like I was levitating off the couch. Looking back, I'd peg this as the moment when I decided I wanted to become a priestess like them, with their rituals and prayers and burials, their fire and food. But that adventure was still a ways away.

Jody, who'd been standing next to us with both hands raised, evangelical-style, to receive information, lowered them. "As an energy healer, I can tell you that your work is done."

"You've found your *tikkun* path," said Ellie, kneeling by her bag like a postulant to pack up her flutes.

Rabbi Rayzel touched me on the arm and said, "*Tikkun* means repair, Kass. It's a Jewish term. *Tikkun olam* means to heal the world. You healed around your own abortion to help repair the world."

Dang. To think that three years ago I was just a "Rock-Bottom Loser Entertaining Offers from Several Religions."

Shoshana, long sand curls flowing over her loose floral shirt, walked over to me and fanned a deck of collage tarot cards that she had made. (When I asked Rayzel about the link to Judaism, she replied, in true entrepreneurial Rosh Hodesh form, "We're creating the market.") "Pick one," Shoshana told me. At random, I picked a glossy five-by-three card and turned it over. A woman's feet were running across the sky above a fierce blue ocean.

"Ohhhh!!!" Shoshana clapped her hands. "If I could have picked a card for you, I would have picked that one!"

"What does the card mean?" I asked, matching her excitement. A water theme had been present in each ritual for abortion: water baby, Living Water, *mikveh* and Miriam's Well, even the Midwife for the Soul had instructed me to "inhale the waves."

"The only constant of water is that it moves," said Shoshana. "The woman on the card is going someplace. You're going someplace. I don't know where you're going, but you're on your way."

Ten minutes later, Rabbi Rayzel and I arrived at the train station in her minivan. "You're going to need seven days to let the dust settle," she told me. "And then your life is going to take off."

17

TRAVELS WITH ABORTION MONEY

EIGHT YEARS AND TWO MONTHS AFTERWARD—I took a train home, and my life fell apart.

Greg stood in my office doorway, appearing gaunt, his face drawn. "I'm thinking I can stay in a hotel while we do couples therapy. Or, we can call it." He stared at me, rubbing the back of his graying head, asking me to make the decision about our five-year relationship.

"Let's call it," I heard myself say.

I had promised him that I would return to Austin with him when my graduate program ended. I had believed I would want to do that when the time came. My graduate program had ended. I wanted to want to go. But I didn't want to go.

We had fought. We had each pleaded with the other to change their mind. During a shouting match about moving, he ripped off his shirt like Hulk Hogan. I'd cried in the porta potty at a wedding. The couples' therapist he mentioned had outlined our irreconcilable plans—he wanted a vegetable garden in Austin, I wanted to live in Manhattan and die there. I wanted my ashes scattered up and down the avenues. We had an idea to buy an Airstream and drive across the United States until one of us conceded to a permanent geographical sacrifice.

Instead, Greg and I took turns carrying moving boxes to the street and loading them in a rented minivan parked in front of our building. I placed two dog bowls on the backseat for Bug, the grief beagle whose loss I'd be grieving now. He tugged on a leash that I'd looped around my wrist. I picked him up, and he wiggled and howled until at last I set him down on a towel. This new, healed version of myself had done all the talking for me, had given full custody of my dog to my ex and the vast Hill Country of Austin, where Bug could run his beagle legs. Reaching through the window, I played with Bug's long ears, soft as pads of moss, and kissed his head. Greg and I hugged and apologized. I watched the silver minivan ease into traffic. I wouldn't see them again.

I walked inside alone and collapsed on the bed and had a long biblical cry.

"You'll look back on this as one of the biggest losses of your life," said older friend of mine, who was weeping vicariously over the phone. There were times when I felt so heavy I couldn't stand up, as though all my clothes were made of lead.

At twenty-eight, I was the same age as my mother when she gave birth to me. I considered it a strong possibility that I would never have children. Not quite sure what to do with myself, in the weeks after Greg and Bug took off, not sure what to want or what to feel, I noticed the fine lines shooting around my eyes like rays and went online to order a tube of La Mer eye cream the size of my pinky finger.

At my age, my mother had been married to my father for four years and adopted a cocker spaniel. I, on the other hand, had moved in with two boyfriends, bought furniture, adopted animals, and then had mini-divorces. Many people in my generation are children of true divorce who prefer to do a pilot run "marriage," raising surrogate babies, such as plants and animals, before advancing to a formal agreement involving aspirational words and phrases such as "forever" and "until death do us part." But I saw through my attempts to buck the patriarchy and play it cool. I wanted to marry, and I feared I had missed all my chances.

Three weeks after Greg and Bug left, I sat down in my office and opened an email: it was my landlord, evicting me via email. I had to leave and I had nowhere to go. A couple of days later, another email: my teaching contract wouldn't be renewed because of bureaucracy regarding my graduation date. Boyfriend, dog, apartment, job. Gone.

According to a great many spiritual teachers, it's pretty normal for a person to lose the life they know in order to rebuild on a sturdier foundation. So perhaps I could have expected a cosmic hurricane to shake my life so mercilessly that it would come apart and be impossible to put back together again in any recognizable form.

"Don't worry," my mother said, over the phone. "The universe has a plan."

By "universe," I was almost positive the she was referring to herself.

She invited me to move back home with her.

"You still have the abortion money to buy your plane ticket home, right?"

"Yes," I replied.

I wept while I washed dishes, stripped the bed, and sold furniture. I took the translucent bottle emblazoned with the gold cross, the Living Water, off of my windowsill and put it into a shoebox. Guiding Light's flag went next. The altar was inside of me now.

Friends came over to say goodbye, and then nearly every one of them scattered across the globe for marriages, careers, and fellowships. I was single, broke, unemployed, uninsured, and moving home to my mother's house at the age of twenty-eight.

I APPLIED A COAT OF GLOSS to my lips in the bathroom at Joseph Beth Café in Lexington, Kentucky. I raked a brush through my hair, parting it down the middle. My mother's hairdresser had "turned on the lights" and made me blonder and the dark streak blacker. In the restaurant, Will-B was waiting by the hostess stand. The sleeves of his white T-shirt were rolled up. His knee-high rubber boots were splattered to muddy perfection. I had come to let him go.

Releasing him had been an unusual decision to make, since he wasn't exactly begging me to come back. Still, it took two years. I ran it past a trusted counselor of mine. I wanted to see whether letting him go without confessing love would work. I wanted a new relationship, just one, just once, that wasn't haunted by thoughts of him.

Will-B had a girlfriend of three years, whom he started dating five days after the last email he had sent me. They lived together in the house he bought. I think they had a cat. I waved at him like a dork. His eyes softened as he took off his baseball cap. My mouth went dry. I may or may not have been visibly shaking.

A waitress plunked two glasses of water and two sandwiches on the table. I had typed my script on a piece of paper that I pulled out of my back pocket and unfolded.

"Sorry this is so formal," I said, tucking my hair behind my ear.

Will-B chuckled, scrunching up his nose. "Don't worry. You can't mess up."

"Well, I did mess up. Pretty bad. And I'm really sorry. I realize this happened nearly nine years ago. Maybe you don't think of it at all anymore, but I think about it and you every day. So I'm here to make amends." He tendered a deep nod. I read out loud: "I consciously withdrew affection from you when you were in Korea. I knowingly put myself in the position to betray you. I rerouted the course of our relationship and our lives. I knew I was hurting you when I quit answering your phone calls and gave you a weak explanation. When you came to Vermont, I sent you mixed signals and then set you up to have to meet Noah. Being a drunk college kid did not give me the right to violate a commitment or to treat you like that. I knew I was making the wrong choices with you and I made them anyway. If I could go back in time, I would never have put myself in a position to violate your trust in the first place. I would have shown up at the airport. I loved you. I love you."

When I broke away from the page, his eyes were waiting to meet mine.

"I feel the same things you do," Will-B said.

I wanted to know what he meant and how he meant it, but I had wired my brain to let him go today. He was staring at me with an unnerving green-brown gaze, and I was cowering in my seat.

One drunken mistake had spun me out into the atmosphere. It took me nine years to get back, though I wasn't back yet—or I was, but I wanted to be better.

"I still have the letter you left in Vermont," I told him. He smiled reluctantly. "I know I'm nine years late, but here's my reply. You said that you couldn't give me happiness, but you could, because you did. You were an incredible friend to me. You would call me out of the blue when I was sad. You said I didn't want a guy like you, but my boyfriends have been approximations of you. I actively looked for the Will-B in them. Don't tell them I told you that."

"I've had the same email account since 1999," he said. "When you asked me to meet you here, I read through our old emails. I want to apologize if I ever hurt you."

"Thanks," I said, wondering how he thought he might have hurt me.

I could hear my mother telling me, "Now, Kass, you know it's not fair to expect him to say anything back when your offenses were clearly much worse," but I did want an apology. I wanted him to tell me he had consciously left the relationship murky throughout high school and in college and when he came to Vermont and when he kept showing up in Kentucky and New York because of his feelings for me and to confirm that it wasn't all in my head.

"You tried to erase me from your memory with that loser in Vermont and then you dated guys you found similar to me," Will-B said, looking me dead in the eye with a neutral expression. I tried not to flinch.

"Strong psychoanalysis," I said. I ripped a drag from my water glass, hydrating for the last lap. One more thing I wanted to say.

"I question the logic of wanting to be with someone I haven't really known in years, but I still do want to be with you. So this is probably going to sound kind of absurd—"

"I bet it won't," he said.

"I am letting you go," I said, applying pressure as though each word were a key on a piano. "I'm letting go of the idea that we will ever be together, now or when we are a hundred and twenty. Do not look for me in heaven or purgatory or hell or wherever we go after this. We're not doing this in the next life. I cannot go through this again."

He furrowed his brows, full of an emotion I couldn't decode. "I mean, goddamn, yeah," he said, letting his accent take over, raising his voice to a volume the bartender could hear about ten yards away, "if we haven't figured it out by now, then yeah, why would it work later?"

"Was there something else you wish I had said?" I asked.

"Yeah. Same thing we're always hoping we're going to say," he said. Again, I wanted x-ray vision of his brain to understand what he was implying, but I had just said the words I had spent two years (or fourteen?) preparing to speak out loud to his face. I didn't feel resolved around Will-B, but I felt straightened out with myself.

Out in the parking lot, behind my pickup truck, we turned to face each other. Pushing thirty now, he had faint crow's feet, same thick eyebrows. I wrapped my arms around his neck, heart thumping so hard I worried he could feel it. He hugged me back and kissed my cheek. I resisted the urge to turn and kiss him on the mouth.

I installed myself in the driver's seat and promised myself that I wouldn't let the first boy who ever broke up with me, the high school fling, the person I loved when I got knocked up, this irresistible hometown motherf*cker, to weaken my capacity to love someone else. I started the engine while he headed the other way jingling his car keys by his side. I wanted him to turn around, but in my rearview mirror, he was gone.

III.
LOVE
ON
EARTH

- 18 -

THE ENLIGHTENED F*CK

EIGHT YEARS AND EIGHT MONTHS AFTERWARD—I lay alone on my black bedcovers, flipping through *Fear of Flying* before I dressed for the evening. This book had been my sex Bible, its underlined passages like time capsules of my slow and ongoing zipless awakening. But there was no such thing as a zipless f*ck. No such thing as unemotional sex without further solicitations, not for me. My quasi-zipless escapade went like this: I cheated on the guy I thought I would marry. I drank and drank and broke promises to others and myself and got pregnant and had an abortion partly out of fear and partly out of love. Nightmares came, regrets came, sorrows came, even while I enjoyed the privilege to pursue my education, a "career," and unfettered meditation and prayer. Still, I had to heal more. Zipless means "passionate." The glory wasn't in the zipless f*cking. The glory was in the zipless seeking.

As much as I wanted to draw the stage curtain on the story of my abortion, the story wasn't over yet. It was time to "rededicate to the temple." Get some sexual healing. My mom had gotten more action than I had in the past couple of years.

Speeding toward my twenty-ninth year on earth, I found that Isadora Wing and I had more in common than a wandering eye. Like my attempt at a zipless f*ck, Isadora's left her miserable and dissatisfied, emancipated and triumphant, all at the same time.

I had just moved to a new apartment in Manhattan with low ceilings and no closet. The exposed balance rod on which I had hung my clothes had buckled and snapped in two, in the shape of a V, the clothes sliding down, forming a sad valley on the left wall of my room. I was currently staring at it from the bed, mustering the energy to put down my former sex Bible and sift through the pile to pick out a getup for tonight, even though I was sure I'd wear a green dress.

I left *Fear of Flying* on my bed and sat on the stool at my round vanity mirror, with a damp towel wrapped around me, and dusted a powder brush on my forehead in preparation for a date. I hadn't been on a first date in five years. I wasn't sure I remembered how to kiss, let alone do anything else, but I had wanted to kiss this person for a long time.

I HAD FIRST NOTICED HIM DANCING on a table at Columbia's winter ball two years earlier, when I was still with Greg. Wearing a black tutu of a dress, I'd been leaning against the buffet table, trying not to get caught stealing a glance. I held a paper plate and gorged myself with pita bread and green olives. Greg was sitting in one of the chairs lined up against the wall, talking to a poet in a giant pink polka-dotted bowtie, because he didn't dance. I wanted to dance so badly I thought I'd spontaneously combust in a ball of prancing flames. In a navy blue blazer and red tie, surrounded by a cheering crowd, the dancing man lifted the heels of his brown construction boots and moonwalked across the table while everyone screamed and shouted. I started laughing. He and I had made eye contact for a moment, or at least I thought we had, and then he returned his attention back to his screaming fans.

The following year, we ended up sitting next to each other on a bus leaving Manhattan. I was overheated and out of breath after a run through the terminal halls, the sleeves of my black jacket rolled up by the time I collapsed in the seat next to him. I stopped fanning myself and reached out to shake his hand as an excuse to touch him.

"Kassi Underwood," I said.

"I'm Mike Murphy," he said. Judging by the name and wicked accent, I pegged him for an Irish Catholic from Boston. He acted shy, but I knew better.

"Glad to meet you," he said, still holding my hand. He had longish, blondish hair and a boyish face. He looked like Tim Riggins, my crush from *Friday Night Lights,* the gorgeous, brooding, emotionally damaged quarterback played by Taylor Kitsch. Within minutes, Mike and I pieced together how many other times we could have met before.

You spend ten years walking the same streets in the same cities. You both move to Vermont at age eighteen, live one hundred yards apart, sit in the same undergraduate classes (different sections), and walk across the same stage at graduation. You don't meet.

You both move to New York to start the same graduate program and take the same classes again (different sections). He sees you in the hallway in a black bomber jacket. You see him dancing on a table. You still don't meet.

Then you board a bus headed to Jersey.

"Do you think it's odd for two people to follow each other around for a decade without encountering each other?" I asked, testing him to see whether he was drawing the same significant conclusions I was. The bus juddered to a stop in a small town of literary acclaim, where we were headed to the same party.

"I can think of weirder," he said, looking at me out of the corner of his eye. Maybe if I'd been single, he would've asked for my number.

ANOTHER YEAR ZOOMED BY BEFORE HE called me on the old-fashioned telephone and asked me on an old-fashioned date, scheduled for tonight. I'd mentioned to him that I was vegan at some point and so, impressively, very impressively, he'd researched vegan restaurants and then called me and told me he was taking me to one. The only other Catholic I'd dated told me his parents wouldn't have accepted me, citing the abortion. But I wouldn't be able to avoid the subject with Mike—because Aspen Baker of pro-voice had invited me and four other women to hit the road, traveling the country to talk about our abortions with rooms full of strangers. I was beyond excited to meet them: Kate Hindman, Mayah Frank, Natalia Koss-Vallejo, and Ronak Dave. I considered this my last and final chance to create the gatherings I imagined. I was flying out to the Bay Area in six weeks to lay eyes on the gals for the first time and get trained for the tour.

Fear of Flying was first published in 1973, the same year abortion was legalized. The zipless encounter was in part an attempt to prevent heartache. I liked to tell myself I had never been dumped—except by Will-B when I was fourteen—but that was only true because I made sure nobody had the chance. I had two-timed Will-B before he could break my heart again; Noah was in the grips of heroin and lacked the focus to break up with me; and with Greg, I had what amounted to a deep and meaningful live-in friendship in which we shared a dog. All attempts to avoid pain had resulted in greater heartache (and one water baby). So I decided to revamp the zipless encounter for myself, creating an aspirational philosophy to guide my future encounters.

The Enlightened F*ck was, above all, an attitude of focused attention and complete trust. I had found that the major component of a sexual experience occurred inside the mind, well before "underwear blew off like dandelion fluff." The E.F. was personal and individual, a f*ck I designed for myself—and it looked like boundless, dauntless, no-holds-barred love. Obviously, this meant no games, no inhibitions, no waiting a certain number of minutes before I texted him back to mask my enthusiasm. It meant not just risking rejection but embracing rejection. Because the entire point of the E.F. is to give without the expectation of getting, without mentally planning the wedding before the salad arrives, without sizing up a person's long-term spouse potential within the first conversation, without asking him to fill my bottomless void of need. It meant rejecting the advice of many well-meaning therapists and *not* trying to "get my needs met." I would try to meet needs instead. From what I had gathered, human needs were simple: having their views respected, being loved, appreciated, and trusted. Having an adequate supply of water, food, and shelter. And a shitload of fun. I didn't have to generate some kind of fun feeling and then theatrically show it off. Actually, being this person meant being natural. The E.F. meant letting a man be free and letting myself be free, too.

It would take a lot of meditation. A lot of prayer. Constant willingness to shift my perception from trying to get attention, commitment, reassurance, to trying to give it.

Enlightened f*cking may cause orgasm. May cause heartbreak. May cause children. May cause abortion. May cause friendship. May cause love.

But it wasn't my business what came next. What mattered was that I contributed to Mike Murphy's evening with devoted attention, human-to-human, concerned more with what I brought to the encounter than with what I took away from it.

So here I was getting ready for my first-first date in a long time. I reached into the clothes pile and tugged out a long-sleeved stretchy green dress. I shimmied into it and smoothed it out. I pulled on my cowgirl boots by the front door. For this next spiritual experiment, I would be open to making a complete ass of myself.

———————

"I WORK WITH KIDS," MIKE TOLD ME, dipping a soy "chicken" finger into barbecue sauce at a small table. Burly and muscular, he clashed with the restaurant, a vegan soul food place called Red Bamboo in the West Village. "I've run an after-school program for the past five years."

I am going to marry this guy, I thought while Mike talked, revealing a tiny chip in his front tooth. *Woah cowgirl. There you go again. Bring it in. Enlightened f*ck this situation.* After my accidental celibacy, I worried I was emitting desperate "sleep with me" vibes. But I'd meditated. I'd prayed. And I'd let the bush grow wild as a defense against his advances.

"So why did you become a vegan?" Mike asked. "Or is it vegàn?" he joked, pronouncing it as though it were a French word, so it rhymed with "be-gone."

"Why? Do you hate the food here?" I asked cheerfully, avoiding the question. I didn't want to divulge that I became a vegan to make amends to my water baby. Wasn't sure how that one would go over.

"It's delicious," Mike said, examining the faux chicken finger. "I'm gonna cut meat from my diet, starting tonight."

I sat back in my seat. "Six foot two Irish Catholic Boston boy. Recovered bar fighter and ex-booze bag. You eat street meat and roast beef. You're not going vegetarian," I said.

"Yeah. I totally am."

"What for?"

"You."

"You're not quitting meat for me. It's our first date."

"Ms. Underwood," he fake-snapped, locking eyes with me. "Don't tell me what to do."

We bobbed up to the sidewalk a couple of hours later, streetlamps lit overhead. Two men who must have worked at the restaurant heaved trash bags into a Dumpster. I overheard one of them say, "I believe it was Machiavelli who made reading books an event in the evening by putting on the robes of the court."

I burst out laughing. Then Mike grabbed me right in the middle of my laugh and kissed me.

"I like you," I said, wishing he would kiss me again. Without further conversation, we turned back toward the sidewalk hand in hand and carried on in the dim light. The winter branches hung over the sidewalk, their shadows overlapping. Holding hands with him, I felt like we were two innocent teenagers. Then, Mike proposed that we retire to his apartment in Queens.

For what? I wondered. Sex? On the first date? I was offended.

But not that offended. He had a Rolling Stones poster on the wall and floral sheets on the bed. Pictures that the kids in his after-school program had drawn were taped up on each side of his desk. His laptop was wrapped in a dishtowel printed with the words "God Bless America."

"Let's take off our shoes," Mike said, with a conspiratorial lift of the eyebrows. I wasn't sure what he was up to. We sat side-by-side on the edge of the bed; he leaned down to untie the laces of his brown Steel Toes, and I nervously pulled off my boots. My palms were damp. I wanted to be all uninhibited and cool, but my nerves had me locked up.

"What's with the dishrag?" I asked, pointing to his computer.

"Just keeping it warm," Mike said, his back to me, leaning over his desk to type on his computer. "What, you don't protect your computer with a dishrag?" he asked, still typing.

"You Can't Hurry Love" by The Supremes blared out of the two small speakers flanking his computer. Mike reached out and offered me his hand, spinning me across the hardwood floor behind his bed, then he had me spin him, which made me laugh. Then he curled his hand into a fist, whipping it in a circle, his signature move: "The Liquorish Whip." I did the flapper dance. The dance party carried on as we jumped on the bed and he busted out the Robot, mechanically twisting and moving his arms. He grabbed me by the waist and pulled me in for another kiss.

I unbuttoned his shirt and peeled it off of him. Eight tattoos— some had been needled in the middle of the night using equipment available at any Rite Aid. He had the body of a guy with a five-hour workday and a leisurely writing schedule who spent the rest of his time lifting free weights in the kitchen and bombing his bike around the city.

He hovered over me with his muscles and tattoos and unruly hair and I gave in at 4 A.M.

The next morning, my dress and tights lay in a crumpled pile beside the bed. Mike was off to work with the kids. I dizzily gathered my clothes from the floor and dressed. I sipped a cup of coffee—he'd memorized my drink order when we had stopped by Starbucks the night before and picked me up a soy no-foam latte before he left for work—and I wondered whether he would ever call me ever again.

Days passed. He did not call me. I jogged through the city and had a girls' night in Brooklyn, keeping my phone on my person at all times. But I still did not hear from Mike.

At home in my apartment, I knelt down before my meditation cushion and asked God to remove my fear and remembered there was no such thing as rejection and humiliation if I had no grabby motives. Then I sat down on my meditation cushion. I closed my eyes and visualized Mike standing in front of me. I put my hands on his shoulders and looked him dead in the eye, and I told him that I hoped he would find enlightened f*cks with someone, even if it weren't with me. If he never wanted to call me again, then he was more than welcome to be free.

Then, I texted Mike and invited him to my apartment. He jumped on his bike and pedaled over with no helmet and no brakes and stayed for forty-eight hours. He took off his green cable-knit sweater, transforming his literary snob getup into a look that mocked pretense: a stained Budweiser shirt with the sleeves cut off. He was a vegetarian writer who prayed to God and played bass guitar in a death metal band and worked with children and almost flunked out of college and had an Ivy League degree. He was everything. I let him know. Between sessions, we lay in bed sideways, facing each other, as he stroked my hair and told me about what he'd been up to for the past ten years.

After college graduation, Mike had moved back to his hometown on the ocean in Beverly, Massachusetts. I had been there once before, when I was pregnant and extremely sick with nausea. Noah had taken me—we'd stayed over with a childhood friend of Mike's, of all people.

Mike's father, a former professional hockey player, saw his son wasting time and turning into one of the fabled local drunks, when he knew that Mike was meant to be a writer. So he sat Mike down and then sent him away from the place where he had grown up.

Mike showed up in Times Square with nothing but $400 in his pocket. He landed a job running an after-school program the same day he interviewed and started grinding out his application to Columbia's writing program. He was sitting in his office one day, kids racing around his desk, when his older brother called. His father had died suddenly of a heart attack. Mike was twenty-four. Numb and disoriented, he forged ahead and mailed his materials to Columbia, wishing he could have told his father the news when he was accepted.

"I'm so sorry," I told him. I knew there was nothing I could say to make his father's death better. I knew nothing would. I had no idea what losing a parent felt like, but after grieving the unlived life of what might have been my first child, I could listen to someone talk about an inconceivable void without needing to try and fix it.

"My dad always told me to marry a girl named Kassi," Mike said, ramping up his accent.

"Stop it," I said. He took a grape from the fruit plate wedged between us, looking like a statue of Dionysus, wavy hair and all. No way his father told him to marry a girl by my name. Plus, no man brings up marriage on the second "date." Greg hadn't said the M-word in five years, except metaphorically: "I'm not 'married' to eating Chinese food for dinner."

"I'm serious. He'd say, 'Hey Mikey, I'll buy you a house if you marry Kassi.'"

"But how would he—?"

"Kassi was the name of a girl who lived down the street when I was a kid. But my dad would tell me I was going to marry Kassi."

"That is weird," I said, curious as to what he was getting at.

"Hey. I read your story in the *New York Times*," Mike said.

This is when I learned that publishing my story about my ex-pregnancy for a readership of millions had removed the need to tell Mike about it in a disclosure with some degree of formality. He continued, "So I looked up Noah on Facebook."

Noah had been convicted most recently for stealing packages of beef from a grocery store and shut away in prison. I held him in my prayers, not because I felt smugly superior and took pity on him or anything, but because we had the same soul sickness, and he had fathered my mini-baby, plus he had a daughter whom the sickness didn't want him to raise. I didn't want to have to defend Noah to Mike. I blinked and waited.

"I know people who know him," Mike said. "I bet I woulda been buddies with him if I'd known him." I was relieved. "But if you and I had met when we were in college, and it had been me and not him, I hope I would have figured out a way to keep the baby."

"How Catholic are you?" I asked him, sincerely not sure what he was trying to convey.

"I was an altar boy for eight years, but now I go to church only for weddings and funerals. This isn't a religious comment. Let me rephrase it. If that had happened to us, I like to think I would have said something to the effect of, I'm not afraid of abortion, adoption, or a baby."

His salesman quality was awfully funny in this context. He'd also memorized all 150 names of the children in his afterschool program. I'd overheard him talking to parents off-hours and seen him on the computer, outwitting the public funding system to sneak kids into his program for free. I was comforted that all three options could be legitimately available.

"Would you have given me your input?" I asked. "Because I would have wanted it."

"We would have explored the options thoroughly," he said.

I hadn't expected us ever to explore the options. I had an IUD, the most effective form of birth control next to abstinence. But, a month later, I could tell something was off in the nether regions. My gynecologist sent me for an ultrasound to have my IUD placement checked.

IN MY BEDROOM, I TOSSED CLOTHES into my orange bag, packing to meet the pro-voice girls in California. I recited their names in my head: Kate, Mayah, Natalia, Ronak. I pitched jeans in the bag. Razor, novels, cowgirl boots, blue tube socks blessed by Hebrew priestesses.

My phone buzzed on the vanity. It was a private number.

"Hello?" I said.

It was my gynecologist, calling two weeks after my ultrasound, to tell me that the results showed my IUD had slipped out of place. My birth control had stopped working.

Twenty minutes later, I had my heels jammed in the stirrups at her office to have the useless IUD removed. Since Greg and I hadn't really tested the IUD in recent years, I had no idea how long ago it had fallen.

As she plugged my records into the computer, the doctor told me absently that she had called in a prescription for Plan B, sometimes called the "morning-after pill," at the pharmacy. (It's over-the-counter now, but it was prescription-only at the time.) My feet dangled off the edge of the exam table.

"I can't believe I'm saying this," I said, "but I'm not sure I'll take it."

"Why?" she asked, incredulous that I, a late-twenties woman whose birth control had failed, would hesitate to take a miraculous drug that would save me from pregnancy with a man I had been dating for only a few weeks.

"I have no idea," I lied, embarrassed to tell the truth. I had nothing but positive feelings toward Plan B as backup birth control. But with this particular partner and this particular malfunction, a voice at the core of me objected to the idea of taking the tablet.

I picked up the prescription anyway and put the packet in my handbag. My flight to San Francisco would depart in the morning. With an embarrassment of luggage, I rode the subway to Mike's place. He met me at the train stop and carried my luggage three blocks to his building. In his room, he had cold cans of Diet Coke and two slices of vegan cake on the bed.

"I don't want to alarm you," I told him, as I tossed my Plan B into the buffet of baked goods and sat down, "but there's a slight possibility I am 'with child.'" I explained the inner-workings of my T-shaped nonhormonal birth control that had been placed in my uterus six years earlier.

Mike examined the box, and the two round white pills. To let nature take its course or not? That was the question.

"Are you able to take Plan B, after—?"

"Yes," I replied. "No long-term effects on the lady business."

The doctor had showed me the ultrasound of my eggs, piled high in my ovaries like grapes, plenty of half-Underwoods for later. Mike and I faced each other on the bed, seated cross-legged. A glum expression washed over him at the prospect of my taking the morning-after pill (or, in my case, the two weeks–later pill—Plan B is supposed to be taken within seventy-two hours after the birth control failed, but my doctor prescribed it anyway, just in case it might work to prevent another pregnancy). Had Mike never encountered this problem before?

"Do you think it'll upset you to take it?" he asked, preparing a forkful of cake. "I don't want you to feel bad."

"Do you think it'll upset *you*?"

He scanned the box, turning it over, searching for a reason for me not to take the pills.

"I could take on a second after-school program and put you on my insurance policy. Two master's degrees from Columbia—a baby's seen worse."

"It's not like I'm definitely carrying a li'l Murphy-Underwood," I reminded him.

"What do you think about the name Sea Wizard?" Mike said, taking a bite of cake.

"I like it alright, but I kind of had my heart set on Ghostface Jesus."

I popped the pill in my mouth and swallowed.

THE NEXT EVENING, I STOOD ON the street in San Francisco, staring up at a house with tears of gratitude messing up my makeup. I was twenty-eight. The house was a Painted Lady, a sea green Victorian of the style featured on the opening credits of *Full House*. Inside the house was the fulfillment of a wish I'd had when I was nineteen—an in-person gathering for the purpose of talking about our abortions. I carried my luggage up the wide and curving staircase, my head filled with exclamation points. The digs were so nice, it was astounding to remember that, in many regions of the nation and the world, women who have experienced abortion are considered the dregs of society. There, in the doorway, stood four women. I had never met them before, but we had a reunion vibe going on. Ronak, Kate, Mayah, and Natalia.

"Kassi!" said Kate, pronouncing my name *Kass-ay*.

"Yes-s-s-s. The *New York Times* abortion star is here," said Natalia in an announcer voice.

"Abortion superhero, Natalia Koss-Vallejo," I sang back to her.

We weren't saying the word "abortion" freely because we took the word lightly. We were saying the word "abortion" because we could.

An hour later, the living room was strewn with to-go food containers, wine glasses, and cans of Diet Coke, and we were sitting in a sloppy circle. Mayah kicked up on the bed in the living room next to Natalia's chair. I took the couch, squeezing between Ronak and Kate, eager to know their backstories.

"So I was seventeen. Sitting in my pediatrician's office. Cartoon wallpaper featuring Disney characters, the whole nine." This was Natalia, twenty-seven, wearing a silver septum ring in her nose and a peroxide blonde Jean Harlow. She had a midwestern accent, though her mother had emigrated from Colombia. "I'm there for birth control, right, and my doctor tells me I'm already pregnant. According to Wisconsin state law, a minor can't terminate without written consent from her parents. Not old enough to have an abortion, but old enough to become a parent, eh?"

Laughing, Mayah propped her pair of strappy hiking sandals on the coffee table. Her face was a constellation of freckles and shaped like the moon. She leaned over and topped off Natalia's glass of wine.

"Go on, girl," she said, pressing Natalia to continue.

"So I get home and huddle in my closet so my parents can't hear me talking trimesters and cutoff dates with the nurse. I had to get a judicial bypass, which is a fancy way of saying I had to stand in front of a judge and beg an old dude to let me make my own decision."

Natalia passed me a rolled-up copy of *Planned Parenthood Magazine*. I unfurled it and examined her cover photo. She sported a photoshopped superhero cape. I'd watched Natalia on television in a special episode of MTV's "16 and Pregnant" when I was still reeling and unable to imagine returning to normal again, whatever normal was. I certainly never expected that, three years later, "normal" would mean hugging Natalia in a house in San Francisco.

"I was seventeen when I got pregnant, too." Enter Kate, voice from my left, a twenty-year-old blonde Katy Perry double. She had a *what-are-you-stupid* tone straight from Los Angeles. We took turns sticking our hands into the same crinkly bag of potato chips. "The father was older than me and threatened me until I agreed to abort." I wasn't used to hearing the word "father" in this context. Noah came to mind. I wondered whether he considered himself a "father" to our water baby. I wondered whether I was pregnant now, again, whether Plan B had worked, whether I wanted it to work. Part of me hoped it hadn't.

"Day of my appointment," Kate continued, "I'm looking everywhere for a huge sign to come down and tell me to run. No signs. So I'm on the exam table, shaking, crying, hyperventilating, saying, *Okay. Okay. Okay.* I ask the nurses, I say, can somebody hold my hand? But they all hold up their instruments and tell me they all need their hands. So halfway through the procedure, I look up and see this nurse standing above me, wiping my face and neck with tissue. She's wiping my tears, but not holding my hand."

She's wiping my tears, but not holding my hand.

"Afterward," Kate said, "I go to counseling at a crisis pregnancy center in Beverly Hills. I was glad they existed—I'd nowhere else to go—but I felt like this therapy thought abortion was wrong. So I graduate high school and move to San Francisco and start working the lines at Exhale."

"We answer the phones," said a lilting voice that belonged to Ronak, seated to my right. She wore earthy colors, gold, maroon, and navy blue, and had a curtain of glossy black hair. Her grandparents had been freedom fighters with Gandhi in India. "I found out I was pregnant when I was nineteen—ten years ago, and I still remember every detail. Being in my boyfriend's basement apartment with the light shining through the basement window, how his head hung. My culture would never accept a pregnancy out of wedlock. Or an abortion. Women get shamed or shunned. All I wanted was one person to talk to me and tell me I'd be okay. So when I went to the clinic, I didn't know whether I was making the right decision. I just knew that the sleepless nights and hopes for a miraculous miscarriage needed to end. A week after the abortion, the bleeding hadn't stopped—I had to go through the procedure all over again."

"I did, too," Mayah exclaimed. She was lounging back on the bed, holding a glass of red wine. "I got home and I was still pregnant. What the hell is that about?"

"I was diagnosed with PTSD," Ronak replied. "I don't regret my choice—I have no idea what was on the other side of it. But I've never really felt relief about it."

"I was extremely depressed about it for years, but I've never wanted to take it back, either," said Mayah. "I go in for the first procedure—and I'm broke, uneducated, not feeling it with the father, wanting to continue exploring the wilderness." She led whitewater kayaking trips in Portland. "They take me into this small room. Bright lights, bad drugs. They give me an ultrasound. I can't see anything on the screen. The actual procedure was traumatizing. I was so relieved when it was over. Then, same story—I find out I'm still pregnant. So now I start questioning my decision. I get back to the clinic and the ultrasound is a very clear image. I was devastated."

Hearing Natalia, Kate, Ronak, and Mayah tell their stories—harrowing as they were—felt like warm light pouring on my brain. They had no agenda and so they had no fear.

Later, I lay awake on the bottom bunk, my veins sizzling with electricity. It killed me to think that people like us might be lying awake in bed, somewhere else, suffering alone, feeling bound to secrecy or obliged to pledge allegiance to a political persuasion, or numb out psychic pain, or pretend to be sad and regretful if they weren't. Nobody should have to hide the way they feel or police the way they talk about their own abortions. We could call it a baby or a child or an ageless spirit. A fetus or an embryo or the Golden Zygote of the Grand Goddess. We could call them whatever we wanted.

There had never been a more fertile (if you will) opportunity for women to transcend the frequency of all the projections onto a woman—bad mother, selfish, slut, murderer—and be at peace with ourselves and totally untouchable.

The next morning I woke up hearing Natalia say to me: "I had a nightmare we got gunned down on the road for talking about our abortions." I stared at the blurry wall without my glasses, brushing sleep crust off the corner of my eye. So much for untouchable.

"We've just told our stories," she continued, "and then this dude comes in with an AK-47. Everyone's screaming and ducking and running and there's blood all over the chairs and the floor."

"Ever had a prophetic dream before?" I managed, my palms breaking a sweat. I didn't mention it, just kept wiping them off on the sheets.

"I don't think so."

"Then we're probably okay." Not my best logic. "If it makes you feel any better, there's a chance I'm pregnant right now, which would make us a far less exciting target."

Natalia laughed and slid off the top bunk with a gymnast's landing.

Before the tour began, Planned Parenthood, the nation's leading provider of abortions, dropped its "pro-choice" label. It was a powerful act of solidarity with everyone who needed the organization, including the families of protesters and lawmakers who fought to shut its doors. I hoped all the people who needed us would find us—because I needed them, too.

I STOOD IN FRONT OF A bathroom mirror, rubbing Aquaphor into a fresh tattoo on my left biceps. My mother would hate it. All throughout my twenties, I resisted acting on my ink impulses to honor her wish that I would have pristine skin in a wedding dress, but I was twenty-eight and interested in marriage but not so much in wedding dresses, and so I had a tattoo artist illustrate two black pigeons kissing beak-to-beak on my arm. Mike was in San Francisco now, too, and got a matching tattoo on his chest with my name printed in tiny black capital letters next to the smaller pigeon. We'd been dating for two months.

In the other room of the dayglow-splattered bungalow we'd rented, Mike clasped his hands behind his head, staring up at the mirror on the ceiling. I closed the lid on the jar of Aquaphor and sidled up next to Mike on the bed, letting him know that my period had come.

HARDCORE FEMINIST TEXAS CHURCH LADIES

NINE YEARS AND SEVEN MONTHS AFTERWARD. It was 3 A.M. I bolted upright in a panic about the Texas leg of the tour. "They deserve what's coming to them," an Austin man had commented on a Facebook post advertising the tour. His profile photo was a snapshot of a hand (*his* hand?) holding a pistol over a Bible, dredging up memories of Dr. George Tiller, the abortion provider shot in his church in Kansas, plus the homemade bomb left on the front porch of a woodsy health clinic a couple of miles from my studio when I'd lived in Austin. Our caravan of misfit peacemakers would head south in two weeks. What was coming to us, exactly?

Mike made little *pfff* sleeping noises beside me. I reached to the floor, fumbling around until I found my iPhone and switched on the flashlight, following the white beam to the kitchen table. I opened my laptop, thinking of Natalia's nightmare.

I would love to report that I had achieved "nonviolence," quelled my fear and my defenselessness and boldly chose to see peace instead, but my imagination played a reel of all the ways this stranger without a face could barge into a speaking venue and gun us down.

I messaged my Facebook pal who had posted the tour date: "What's this guy's history?"

"Mental illness and addiction," he messaged back. How comforting. "So sorry about this. I'll talk to him," he continued.

I felt mama-bear protective of Natalia, Kate, Ronak, and Mayah. There was no sense in worrying them needlessly if Facebook Man was all talk and no murder. But there was also no sense in risking our lives if a legitimate threat could be intercepted.

The kitchen was dark except for a blade of light from the balcony. I asked Father Google what kind of Texas we were walking into. A battle had begun when politicians passed House Bill 15 in 2011, two years earlier, requiring people seeking abortions within 150 miles of their home to attend a checkup before the appointment: during said checkup, the doctor was required to give her an ultrasound and describe her progeny to her based on a script of inaccurate information written by politicians instead of physicians. Doctors also had to crank up the sound on the fetal heartbeat. People then had to wait twenty-four more hours to obtain an abortion. Neither restriction was medically necessary—in one case, it wasn't even medically accurate.

I slid my eyes across the screen, wondering what all this red tape felt like to the women who wanted and needed abortions. I read an essay that began: "Halfway through my pregnancy, I learned that my baby was ill. Profoundly so." It was titled "We Have No Choice: One Woman's Ordeal with Texas' New Sonogram Law," by Carolyn Jones, a Texas journalist by way of Zimbabwe. She and her husband, parents to a toddler, learned that their unborn boy had spinal and brain defects. "From the moment he was born, my doctor told us, our son would suffer greatly," she wrote. Tears streaming down her face, she was forced by law to stare at her baby, listen to the flicker of his heart while the doctor described his (inaccurate) physical attributes, and then wait twenty-four more hours.

Next came Senate Bill 5, which threatened to ban abortions after twenty weeks and mainly affected situations like Carolyn's. The bill would also require clinics to meet "ambulatory center standards" and to gain "admitting privileges" in a hospital within a thirty-mile radius.

Enforcing "ambulatory center standards" could shut down all but five of the forty-four stand-alone health centers in Texas, home to 5,848,180 women of childbearing age. Only 3 percent of Planned Parenthood's services constituted abortions; the other 97 percent was gynecological health care and prevention. People without insurance— myself included—trusted and relied on these stand-alone clinics for medical services protecting reproductive health.

Like other restrictions, "admitting privileges" were not medically necessary but notoriously difficult to obtain. Catholic hospitals usually declined for religious reasons. Secular hospitals wanted to avoid negative attention, like bombs and gunfire. Hospitals already admitted patients with abortion-related medical emergencies—and such major emergencies were extremely rare, occurring at a rate of 0.23 percent according to a study conducted by ANSIRH. Critics maintained that the mandate was nothing more than a strategy to shut down clinics.

Violence had erupted, too. (That is, in addition to the violence of depriving people of reproductive care.) A man had thrown a bag of Molotov cocktails at State Senator Wendy Davis's office door, and journalists and activists speculated that the motive was related to her reproductive rights activism. In June, I had watched the livestream of Senator Davis's attempt to kill Bill 5 on the Texas Senate floor. Her goal was to talk until she ran down the clock at midnight to delay the vote and thereby keep clinics open. "I'm rising on the floor today to humbly give voice to thousands of Texans who have been ignored," Davis said, with a measured twang, at 11:18 A.M.

Davis had had two abortions. A blonde Harvard warhorse of single motherhood, she talked nonstop during an eleven-hour filibuster on the Senate floor, forbidden to eat, drink water, lean on furniture, or even go to the bathroom. Her pink sneakers became a symbol of standing up.

Crowds hung over the railing that circled in a loop above the Senate floor, cheering for her in burnt orange T-shirts, holding their fists in the air. More than thirteen thousand women had sent Davis their stories to read. She read seven hundred of them out loud. Ellen, raped at age seventeen, wrote: "My only thought was to kill myself, because I didn't know any other option available to me. Thankfully I had a smart, wonderful mother, who took me to have an abortion. The entire experience was horrible, but I cannot imagine what it would be like under the circumstance that Texas now wants to make women undergo. I made a decision to save a life, my own. And it was the most important decision I've ever made."

Davis's filibuster ended at 10:03 P.M., when she was disqualified for going off-topic, but Senate Bill 5 was dead. The room erupted in cheers and applause. But a new piece of legislation, House Bill 2, advanced identical restrictions.

It passed.

Texas had turned into a war zone. I clicked through photographs online. A state trooper pinned an activist's face to the ground, blood puddling around her mouth. Women chained themselves to the Texas Senate railing and were physically dragged away by security. To mock the old-fashioned bill, young women had dressed up in 1950s costumes, sporting short black gloves, tulle hats, and dresses cinched at the waist, looking daggers at the lawmakers.

Tampons were confiscated from purses and handbags at the State Capitol because security guards feared that women gathering on the balcony above the Senate floor would hurl menstrual period plugs at members of the Senate. It was perfectly legal, however, to breeze by the security desk packing a handgun. The right to bear arms in Texas had more constitutional protection than the right not to bear children.

Worried about Facebook Man and his gun, I read the log of violent acts against abortion clinics and reproductive health facilities, all perpetrated by rogue Christians since 1977. It didn't make me feel better. There were thousands of criminal activities, including 8 murders, 17 attempted murders, 182 acts of arson, 42 bombings, and an inventory of other incidents. Doctors rarely stay in the same hotel twice. Being stalked and receiving harassing phone calls were commonplace parts of their jobs. In Nebraska in 1991 an arsonist burned down Dr. Leroy Carhart's farm in a fire that killed his dog, his cat, and his seventeen horses—a letter to his clinic verified that the fire was vengeance for his profession. And the slaying of Dr. George Tiller in his own church continued to weigh on my mind.

All across the United States, the number of legal restrictions like the impositions in Texas had shot up. Way up. Over the course of two years, up to two hundred thousand women in Texas turned to dangerous illegal abortion methods used before *Roe v. Wade,* or taking drugs such as misoprostol or mifepristone. A *New York Times* graph showed a disturbing correlation between the number of abortion restrictions and the number of Google searches for do-it-yourself methods in twenty-five states, including Kentucky—and Texas.

Returning to Austin seemed like time-traveling to an era when abortion was illegal, when women drank bleach and ate black market herbs to deal with an unwanted pregnancy. I closed my laptop and sat in the dark. Texas was the nation's most dangerous place to have an abortion, not just because new restrictions closed clinics and left people to their own DIY devices, but because anyone who got an abortion was now considered lucky. What I didn't know was whether Facebook Man posed a sincere threat.

"Tell somebody," my mother commanded over the phone the next morning. "This is getting scary, Kass."

"I don't want to be melodramatic," I said. I also didn't want to ignore him in case this dude happened to get an idea he couldn't let go of.

"You should have armed security," my mother said. "Or don't go."

After I hung up with my mother, I got down on my knees and prayed for Facebook Man. I didn't really want to pray for him; part of me worried that by praying for him I was implicitly condoning violence (in word or in deed) or leaving myself vulnerable to him. But by the time I was finished, I remembered he was human like me.

The practice of love demands that you see peace where everyone else sees war; even when presented with evidence of war, you must see peace instead. When everyone thinks you're bonkers for staking a claim on peace, see peace anyway. Acknowledge and comfort the suffering, speak out and alleviate the suffering in concrete ways, and ask them to see peace with you. When you cannot see peace because war is everywhere, war and angst and suffering and scarcity and evil, call upon all your superpowers and magic and prayers and arts and rituals and exercises and gods and monsters of love to help you see peace instead.

But also, don't be an idiot.

I stood up and emailed Exhale to request armed security.

CARVING OUT STORYTELLING DENS ABOUT ABORTION, Natalia, Kate, Ronak, Mayah, and I never had a clue what to expect. So far, we'd been surprised and awestruck. In a conservative religious lecture room, a tall Muslim man told us, "I am forever changed. I will now see abortion as a human experience." In a liberal arts classroom, a girl in a cutoff sweatshirt said, "I thought we'd all be yelling at each other. I came in wearing my armor, but it turns out I didn't need it." At one stop, hands shot up and a spontaneous storytelling session emerged, with audience members sharing their experiences with HIV, cystic fibrosis, and divorce. Everybody wants a place to tell the truth without being judged.

Retiring to hotel rooms and crash pads, we ate Chinese food out of to-go containers and watched reality television, amazed by the audiences we had met. But random strangers listening to me talk about my termination had to be helping me way more than it was helping the random strangers. I was a twenty-nine-year-old woman who got knocked up at nineteen, received a blessing disguised as mental torture, and then tried every available method to transform her suffering into enlightenment. I was no ancient master, but I had a spiritual practice that worked for me. The proof was that other people noticed. Once, Mike yelled, "Nothing ever bothers you." Nicest thing anybody had ever said to me.

And recently, a thought had formed in my head with words like skywriting smoke: *Harvard. Divinity. School.* I wasn't Jewish enough to ordain as a Hebrew priestess, but I felt the God in my solar plexus, urging me to become my own kind of priestess.

AUSTIN, TEXAS. 6:15 P.M. Last pro-voice tour stop.

I wandered through a shadowy church courtyard toward a chapel in the Hill Country. I followed behind Kate, who wore platinum hair extensions that flowed down her back. "I want the Second Amendment removed entirely," she announced, pushing open the double-doors of the chapel. Her fingernails were painted gunmetal gray.

I never told my pack about Facebook Man, but I did mistake our armed security guard for a gunman. (In my defense, he was in fact displaying a firearm on his hip.)

A woman was waiting at the end of the chapel hallway with a priestly mantle over her shoulders (though when I looked at photographs of her later, it appeared to be a purple business casual blazer).

Terry was an Episcopal priest. A force. Six feet tall, eyes like flash-lights. She hugged me and I thought, *Whew, okay. Everything is going to be okay.* The first thing I had to know was how she had embarked on the ordination path to priesthood.

Terry and I chatted while the others helped themselves to cookies in a back kitchen. She had a delicate twang. As the story went, Terry thought she was walking into a Twelve Step meeting but instead walked into an Episcopal Bible study—the woman running it invited her in, and the rest, as they say, is a dog collar and an awkward talk with the family.

"What happened when you told your mom?" I asked. (Mom would think I was pranking her if I mentioned the priesthood.) Terry, too, had expected the worst, but her mother took Terry's hands in hers and said, "You will be a good priest."

"Wow," I said, trying to imagine my mother saying that to me, with no luck.

Then I let Terry in on my Harvard Divinity School head buzz. The photos on the homepage pictured Buddhist nuns in maroon robes, Muslim scholars in hijabs, yogis in Lululemon, and atheists in button-down plaid shirts.

I just didn't see how I'd get into *Hah-vahd*. I had earned Ds in high school. I broke down in tears when my college counselor told me my first SAT scores. (I needed approximately four hundred more points before I'd consider my brain to be human rather than broccoli.) More to the point, it was *divinity school.* On my official undergraduate tran-script, I saw evidence of my having earned an A in an Eastern Reli-gions class that I have no memory of taking. Plus, my abortion was in the *New York Times.* I understood the holy motives for ending a pregnancy—and the moral knots in my own—but I wasn't so sure that the virtuous Ivy League religion scholars reading applications would come to the same conclusion.

The last time I had sat through a church service of my own volition, I had been nineteen and pregnant and I couldn't feel God. My prayer temple was the bathroom. My house of worship was everywhere and anywhere on earth: church basements and Rabbi Rayzel's red tent and Immaculate Conception Seminary and the New York Buddhist Church and a motel room in Santa Barbara and Ava Torre-Bueno's office and my bedroom and my mother's house and abortion clinics.

The other problem was Harvard was located in Massachusetts. Why leave New York City when you can just climb into a coffin, lie down, and close the lid?

"I am so excited for you," Terry said, as though I'd already been accepted.

This brought a smile to my face. I said, "If life ever takes me to Massachusetts, I'll apply."

I had nestled into a couch between Ronak and Kate. Across from us sat Terry, a therapist, and a midwife. Aspen had come, too. The square of couches morphed into a circle once we were all together.

"In the '60s, a young woman who cared for me disappeared," Terry told us. Her voice shook with emotion. "I never knew where she went," she continued. Her caretaker had been shipped off to a farm for pregnant girls so the neighbors wouldn't see her growing belly. "I sent her cookies, but I had no idea why she wasn't in my life anymore." Terry tore a tissue from the box on the arm of the couch and wiped her eyes. The war in Texas had brought the trauma back to the fore.

The midwife, wearing a long cotton skirt, began to weep too. She had her hands in her lap, fiddling with her wedding ring, a simple gold band. "When I work with families," she said, "and someone has a very good experience having their baby, I really appreciate knowing, so I want to tell you: I have been married for twenty-eight years. My husband and I have four children. When I had my abortion, we were already married. And we have never sat down and talked about how

I feel about it." She had sugar and fire in her voice. "I want to tell you what you've done. I'm gonna go home and—maybe not tonight—but I'm gonna start a conversation about it. Because my abortion affected me a lot more than I thought."

Terry put her arm around the midwife, pulled her close, and kissed her head.

"I'm not afraid of telling him," the midwife continued. "He's fantastic."

"I bet he's got some things to say to you, too," said Terry.

"I think there's a conversation to be had, not just a story to be told," she said. "The hard things make us closest to each other," she added. "And when you've been married as long as I have, you *look* for those things."

This gave us a chuckle.

"If you don't mind—" Terry addressed the circle. "We pray when we start something and we pray when we finish something. I just can't end this without doing some praying."

A year had ferried by since I first met the girls in San Francisco. I took Kate's hand on my right and Ronak's hand on my left, squeezing them both.

Terry sent us off with this prayer: "Beloved Mother-Father God, we thank you for this time to be in our stories with each other. We thank you for this extraordinary mission. We pray for your care for this community as they go forth. We pray for your guidance for this community so that they can see what is in front of them and know what to do next. Hold us together here and shower us with love and with compassion and send us forth in the world to do good. Amen."

20

SPIRITUALLY BLONDE

NINE YEARS AND EIGHT MONTHS AFTERWARD—The year had been a surreal montage of photo shoots, live television interviews, and star-studded events, all to bring love to people who'd experienced abortion. To think, just four years earlier, I was crouched down on a hot Texas road alone, trying not to feel sad. Now I was heading home to Mike in the neighborhood where we'd moved in together. There he was, jogging toward me with his long hair flowing behind him and his red high-top sneakers slapping the sidewalk.

"Hey babe," I yelled, running toward him, a bag of books slung over my shoulder. We caught up to each other and walked hand in hand, dodging pedestrians.

"What's bothering you, babe?" Mike asked, bringing me out of a blur and back to the street.

"Nothing's bothering me. Big night. Just thinking."

I'd spoken at another event.

"Can you turn it off?"

"I don't want to turn it off."

Fights like this had become commonplace: I worked and traveled all the time; Mike's "love language" is quality time. He enjoyed aimless walks around the neighborhood that lasted from noon until nightfall. I enjoyed work, meditation, dancing, and sex.

"Do you know what I think about all day?" he said.

"Tell me," I said.

He pulled me down a desolate side street and stopped just shy of a streetlamp.

"I think about you. I think about us. I think about earning another grad degree so I can make enough money for the children I want to raise with you."

"Are you freaking out because you're about to turn thirty?" I asked.

"No," he snapped. "Because you're all business, toots. You put up walls and make it impossible to get through to you."

Once the serotonin, norepinephrine, and dopamine of the honeymoon phase wore off, I didn't know how to enlightened f*ck a serious intimate commitment. Relationship problems weren't new to me; though they had morphed into different shapes over the past decade. With Will-B, I dealt by straying and even though he loved me anyway, I didn't have the capacity to receive it; with Noah, the takeaway was, trying to fix someone is not the same as loving them; with Greg, I had a spiritual fitness training ground to work out my neuroses, from jealousy to ungrieved grief. I had learned how to live *with* myself, but I wound up *by* myself.

"We have sex," I said to Mike.

"Sex is not love," he yelled. Then, "I'm sorry I raised my voice."

"What can I do?" I begged.

"Love me! Love me!" he said. "Show me you love me."

He charged back toward Broadway, and I chased after him.

In my journal, I wrote and wrote and wrote without letting my pen stop moving and without judging what I put down on the page.

This is how I discovered my true feelings, even if my head wanted to delude me: writing with pen and paper, nonstop, no thinking, for three pages. It was like an exorcism of my delusions, the lies that made me think a life that wasn't working, was working. It's how I found out I wanted to break up with Greg, even though I loved him. I had to write it to myself in a letter and break the news to myself. I had been shocked: No! But Greg is wonderful.

So I had prepared myself to discover that I wanted to break up with Mike for infringing upon my freedom. Once again, I was wrong about what I thought I wanted. I wrote: *I used to be gentle. I don't want to be the emotionally unavailable addict I become in relationships, always addicted to something. Alcohol, my neuroses, my healing, my work. I want to move to a small town and remember how to be gentle again.*

THREE DAYS BEFORE CHRISTMAS, MIKE AND I rented a chartreuse sedan and headed toward my mother's house, wending from north to south. I was staring out the rain-splattered window when we crossed the Kentucky state line at 2 A.M. Instead of holiday snowflakes, hail from a line of violent storms pelted the windshield. Tornado sirens blared.

The brick house where my mother lived with her husband had a twenty-foot blow-up Santa Claus behind it that we could see from the bottom of the hill. We cruised around until at last Mike killed the engine in the crescent driveway. Rain drizzled down the windshield in thin lines.

Mom leaned out the front door, the cool wind whipping her hair around. A white cotton nightgown billowed behind her.

"Y'all drove down here without a wink between you." Her white cat, Primrose, wove around her bare ankles, and the grandfather clock behind her chimed three times in the foyer. The force of a gale tried to snap the door that she held open, but she held firm.

"Get on up to bed now," she called as we wandered up the staircase.

The next morning, I opened my eyes to a blur: Mike was seated at the edge of the bed, nudging me.

"Kass, wanna go on a hike?" A hike? After a tornado? When we have a hundred errands to run and presents to wrap before Christmas? Where? How? What shoes would I wear?

"Yes," I replied.

Bleary-eyed, I sat on the edge of the bed and pulled on my high-heeled vegetarian cowgirl boots and then went downstairs to have coffee. My mother found me in the kitchen pouring packets of stevia sugar substitute into my mug.

"What on earth are you wearing on your feet?" she asked.

"The only boots I brought," I said.

"You'll slip in those heels," she sang. "Creek's rising."

She plopped down on a kitchen chair and untied her boots. They were pale brown, classic hiking boots. She passed them off to me and I laced them up; they were still warm from her feet.

I opened the door of my mother's pickup truck at the base of a mountain in Berea, a town about twenty minutes south of her house. The wind had teeth. Tornadoes had ravaged the area. Broken tree limbs were scattered across the gravel parking lot like patterns of torchon lace. I stepped into a mud puddle, one hiking boot after the other.

Tree trunks had been pulled up from the earth and tossed on their sides, their roots dangling. I stepped over sticks matted into the mud and logs strewn across the path. The storm had turned the way into a river of amorphous sludge; we could barely discern where the trail ended and the virgin terrain began.

I ran ahead and grabbed Mike's hand and pulled him along. A hound dog raced down the mountain with a man following several yards behind him. Mike and I bent down to pet him; he pawed us with mud.

At last, we circled around by a tree and walked to the edge of the cliff to behold the view, a panoramic swath of my home that was foreign to me, brown and rough and nude from winter. A lake with a name I didn't know twisted through the dead land.

"Kass," Mike said, squaring up to me.

"Yes!" I blurted out preemptively.

He got down on one knee in the mud. He reached into his coat pocket and pulled out a small black box and popped it open.

The ring was bright, Indian gold. It was a snake that coiled around my finger three times and bit its own tail—an ancient ouroboros. On its head sat a blinding diamond. Two emeralds studded its back. They were stones his father had given to his mother when he proposed to her at a stoplight in the 1980s. The ouroboros symbolized regeneration, return, rebirth.

"Yes," I repeated. I stared at the ring as he pushed it onto my finger, turning my hand so the diamond glinted in the sun, curling my fingers into a fist to hide my chipped green fingernails.

MOM AND I HURTLED ALONG a two-lane road in Vermont on a trip to scope out wedding venues. By then, she had emailed me with the subject line: THE WEDDING PLANNER FROM HELL. She had sent reminder emails with bullet lists about the florist. Photographs of her feet in high heels so that I could ditch the wedding heels she hated. Phone calls about why we should honeymoon on a cruise. I suggested we pick dandelions. Go barefoot. Honeymoon in a medically induced "couples' coma."

"The wedding isn't about the bride and groom, honey," said my mother, sitting in the passenger's seat of the rental car, "the wedding is about the mother of the bride."

I laughed and laughed, driving down the open road, but my mother had a point. The wedding was my mother's ritual, the end of our story together and the continuation of her story through me. Cruising wedding venues, Mom and I checked out a summer-camp-type lodge, stayed in an aggressively artsy Brooklyn-infused hipster bed-and-breakfast decorated with obscure tchotchkes, and checked a Vegas-style place with neon blue lights where everybody wore bathrobes. On the second-to-last morning, it was Mother's Day. We sped down the road with sandwiches wrapped in white paper in our laps. Blue police lights flashed from behind.

"Maybe we can lose him." Mom checked the rearview mirror and kept driving.

"Have you seen *Super Troopers*? It's set in Vermont. You're not losing that cop."

"He'll get bored and lose interest."

"Mom, I was once pulled over twice in the same trip in Vermont. There's nobody else out here except people he knows. He sees your out-of-state plates."

She parked on the side of the road and rummaged through her purse in search of her license. The officer was short, burly, and bald. Mom rolled down the window.

"Happy Mother's Day," she said to him, sarcastically.

"Thanks," said the cop.

"What a dick," Mom said, when he walked away to write the ticket.

"Go Mom," I said. "A dick. Wow. I remember when 'heck' was strong language."

"Your mama's getting spicy in her old age," she said.

"Spicy enough to walk me down the aisle?"

My eyes filled with tears. I looked at the dashboard to hide them from her and gulped back the rest of them.

"Well, Kass!" she exclaimed, fanning her face. "I think I'm gonna cry." I rubbed her shoulder and waited for her to accept my invitation. "But no," she said.

No?

"Walking a bride down the aisle is the father's duty. Your father and I are divorced."

I had failed to fully realize that my parents were divorced until I started planning my wedding.

"This is only a halfway Victorian ending, Mama. Dad isn't passing me off to the next man. I would be so honored if you would walk me down the aisle and give me your blessing."

"But your brother's supposed to seat me. You appear in the doorway wearing a white dress. The guests stand up. Wagner's 'Bridal Chorus' goes BAM BAM-BAM-BAM, BAM BAM-BAM-BAM," she sang. "And you walk down the aisle, slowly, on your father's arm."

"Lie back and close your eyes," I said, checking behind us to make sure the cop wasn't watching. I touched her eyelids, leading her in a guided Obliterate-Traditional-Wedding-Expectations Meditation. "I want you to picture all the traditional ways of doing things. Then I want you to picture them fizzling into the ether. I'll be thirty years old when I marry. My tattoo will be visible. I'm not a virgin. I've been pregnant. My abortion clinic's not an hour away from the wedding venue, if the next one works. I've lived in sin with three different men."

"None of whom was the guy who got you pregnant," Mom added. "*Living in Sin with Three Men, Plus a Side Pregnancy with a Random Druggie.* There's a good book title."

"Shhhh," I said. "Eyes closed. Rusty can seat you, but then you can just walk back up to the head of the ceremony. It would mean so much to me if you would walk me down the aisle."

The cop knocked on the window. My mother opened her eyes and rolled it down and he handed her a speeding ticket. As she took the ticket, she wished him a Happy Mother's Day again.

"Fine," she said to me, accepting my invitation.

———————

THAT NIGHT, MY MOTHER AND I were lying side by side in a king-size bed overlooking my wedding venue—a squiggly line of postcard mountains and shadowed valleys.

Weeks after proposing, Mike had been offered a teaching position at a public school in Massachusetts. Which meant, of course, that I had to move. Which meant, of course, that I had to keep my promise to the universe and apply to Harvard Divinity School.

"Mom, I don't know how to tell you this," I said, turning to face her, resting my face in my hand, "so I'll just say it. I'm applying to divinity school." I burst into tears. I felt I'd betrayed her plan for me to become the writer she wasn't. "I'm sorry, Mom. I know you wanted better for me."

"It's not that. I just don't understand why you'd want to lead a church."

I wiped my tears with the sleeve of my jean jacket.

"Lead a *church*? In what, a leopard print leotard and clear heels? No. I just want to understand how other people access the magic of God, or the universe or higher self or reason or Allah or whatever they call it."

"You don't need a Harvard degree to do that."

Bah! Mom and her good points.

I started to list off a litany of reasons why I should apply before I came to the truest one: I didn't know why I was applying to Harvard Divinity School, except that I felt I was supposed to. It would be a financially idiotic decision to attend, and yet, I felt I was supposed to. I'd almost rather die than leave New York, but was going to go with Mike. I had dedicated my twenties to myself; I decided to dedicate my thirties to others.

"It sounds like you're being led, honey," she drawled, rubbing my arm and smiling warmly at me.

MIKE AND I MERGED OUR BOOK collections and donated the doubles. We took turns running up and down three flights of stairs with boxes and dresser drawers and bike parts and lamps and jamming them into a U-Haul hitched to the back of his hunter green SUV. I drove us over the Triborough Bridge without having said goodbye to my friends, in stubborn denial that the move was any more permanent than an extended summer vacation. Waiting in line at the tollbooth, we watched the driver of an SUV swerve toward Mike on the passenger side, and, for no apparent reason, reach out his window and smack the side mirror repeatedly while he shouted obscenities at us. It was a proper New York send-off.

We parked in a sleepy New England town by the sea.

Now—finally—I had time to apply to priestess school.

When I told my friends and my dad that I was applying to Harvard Divinity School, most of them started calling me some variation on the nickname Spiritually Blonde, a la Elle Woods in *Legally Blonde*. I liked it.

Spiritually Blonde: it means staying spiritually dumb. Teachable. A spin off "beginner's mind," a concept in Zen Buddhism that means the mind should be like an empty rice bowl.

And yet, blonde as I am, my mind still had contents. One thing it had was thoughts of Will-B. I dreamt of him, sometimes night after night, even after I had let him go. I wanted to blame my subconscious activity on classic pre-wedding ex-boyfriend dreams, but I'd had recurring dreams of him ever since I was a chain-smoking teenage virgin. Like an invincible kudzu vine, he returned to my dreams, sometimes every single night, sometimes marathon dreams in the same night, for months on end—here I am shaking with fury in front of a green ATM and screaming at him: "I thought we had a deal!"; here we are sitting on top of a long table in an unfurnished white room, discussing the status of the relationship. In one dream he wishes I would come with him, and in another dream, I wish he would stay with me; here we are at a normal party together with a normal life, and then the scene morphs and he treats me like I'm some new acquaintance he has to charm. These dreams preyed upon my unconscious and never stopped.

As the wedding drew near, the dreams of him became daylight thoughts that wouldn't go away. I had an unfinished enlightened f*ck—when I let Will-B go, I had not shown boundless, dauntless, no-holds-barred love. I hadn't been available for rejection. I had stuck with the script to get the job done. I didn't know what to do. One morning at 3 A.M., I sat cross-legged on the carpet in the den with a yellow legal pad on my lap, pouring out an eight-page letter that I had no intention of mailing off—thinking I could drain every last unreserved word I had to say to Will-B from my brain out through my pen. The next morning, I got an email from Will-B's mother. I hadn't spoken to her in ten years. We had never corresponded online before. She wrote that she had visited my website and read my work. "I love the way you write," she told me. I made much of this eerie coincidence, as if her email about my writing were in cosmic conversation with the letter I had just written to her son. I drove to a nearby town and ceremoniously dropped the letter to Will-B in an obscure wastebasket, not sure what to do—enter my marriage with Mike unresolved, or pick up the phone.

21

ROMANTIC PEOPLE IN PARADISE

ELEVEN YEARS AFTERWARD— On a plane to my bridal shower, I heard a little girl say to her brother in the seats in front of me, "Can you find the romantic people in paradise? Can you find them?"

"No," the small boy replied. "Wrong book."

At one of the seven parties leading up to the wedding—oh, to be from the South!—an old friend in my bridal circle gave me the greatest gift: a mason jar of artesian pickles she brought from the West Coast. But that's not all. She let me whisper to her the truth about my thoughts of Will-B—and she listened to me and didn't judge or try to talk me out of my thoughts or appear nervous about having already invested in a bridesmaid dress. She knew Will-B. She had been my housemate in Vermont, with her long black hair and sage wands and windowsills overflowing with greenery. After Will-B and Noah had left, and I was depressed and constantly drunk and felt there was quote-unquote nothing worth living for, she'd lie next to me in my bed and hold my hand and instruct me to close my eyes and picture my life in ten years—and here we were. Eleven years later, actually, holding hands on a couch at my bridal shower.

Then, my old friend gave me yet another great gift. She told me that despite being married to a wonderful man whom we all adored and to whom she was staunchly committed, she was, as it so happened, currently setting an alarm clock and waking up early in the mornings to cry on the bathroom floor, grieving a long-lost sweetheart from ten years past. It was a gift because I realized that I did not want to be a married woman crying on a bathroom floor.

Hard phone calls—and I didn't mean to the florist or the photographer or the rogue wedding planner mom—were part of my preparation for marriage. I was choosing to marry Mike. I wanted to seal off the escape hatch and obliterate the alternative path. (As grief guru Ava might say, picturing the alternative was a defense against grieving. Even a wedding was a choice—and with every choice comes grief.) An underground part of me held out for Will-B.

My rule of prayer: receive no answer? Take no action. Receive an answer: take an action. No answer: no action. Answer: action. I prayed for a solid month: Do I, or do I not, call Will-B VanMeter before I marry Mike Murphy? The same answer came, every single day, for thirty days: yes. Yes, *and* do not give him the power to determine whether I marry Mike.

But what might I say, pray tell? Hey buddy, scale of 1 to 10, how otherworldly would you say our connection was?

The E.F. principles applied here.

Risk everything.

Embrace rejection.

Love big.

My mother's principle applied here, too: "Finish the business."

Fifty-seven days before my wedding date, I picked up the phone.

The pounding in my chest lurched me forward in a gentle rhythm. Faith comes after taking a risk, not before. I had thirty seconds of grief. I had nothing to forgive.

Voicemail.

Here was one possible result: my question answered in one unreturned phone call. But Will-B returned my call the next day. I was frozen and unmoving on a yellow armchair in my den, watching the phone vibrate on the wicker side table. I let it go to voicemail.

I know.

An hour later, I was still curled up in a ball in the armchair like my teenage self, but I was thirty, engaged to another man, a thousand miles from Will-B.

The phone started vibrating again. It was him, calling back. A very bold move usually reserved for mothers, drug dealers, and Twelve Step sponsors.

"Will-B," I sang, as though we had no fraught history.

"Kass." He sounded weary after a morning with horses.

We talked about the weather, the beach, all nonsense and nothing-ness and prologue to this: "Can I ask you something?"

"You don't need my permission to ask me something," he replied.

"When we had lunch a couple of years ago, what did you mean when you said you hoped we'd say the same thing we're always hoping we're going to say?"

He paused for fifteen seconds.

"Kass," he said.

"Okay," I said. I told him I was preparing to marry a person for whom my love was firm, but I had an insistent old thought about him. I acknowledged that my call was perhaps taboo, but I didn't want to turn seventy-five and regret the time I hadn't picked up the phone when I was thirty. I didn't want to turn one hour older and wish I had picked up the phone the hour before. "I can't sit around wondering," I said. "I have this nagging feeling that we were sup-posed to end up together. I can't figure out why it won't go away, no matter how many ways I try to let go. If this isn't a mutual feeling that's exclusive to us, then I need you to break my heart."

He paused again for sixteen years packed into ten seconds.

"I can't say that I have a nagging sensation that we're supposed to be together."

"Okay," I replied.

"Don't you think if God wanted us to be together, we would be?" he asked.

"I think we have free will," I said. "Being together is a choice."

"You don't want to be with me, Kass," Will-B said. "I think you're just trying to rekindle that love and passion and uninhibitedness of childhood."

Sixteen years after we first met, it broke through my dense skull that Will-B was a symbol of my innocent Virgin Mary marriage fantasy. Phone pressed to my ear, I felt faint, struggling to adjust to the discombobulating reality I'd somehow missed.

"Do we need a ritual for closure?" is, remarkably, what *he* asked *me*.

"What would the ritual look like?"

"Maybe I need to tell you to f*ck off. Because we never really officially broke up and told each other to f*ck off."

"By all means," I replied.

"F*CK OFF," he yelled into the phone.

"YOU F*CK OFF," I shouted back.

"Kassi, I love you, and I want you to be happy."

"I love you, too. I want you to be happy, too."

*F*ck off.*

I love you.

I want you to be happy.

The enlightened f*ck was humbling, hilarious, hugely satisfying, and full of the divine kind of love that puts you in your place and somehow draws you closer to all human beings. It was a miracle, grief itself, and it was over. With him, at least.

The next morning, I awoke alone in bed. Disoriented and shaken, I peeled off the damp sheets. I rolled over and reached down to grab my cat eye glasses from the floor. I had lost control of the narrative—missed a crucial element in the plot, been deceived by my own desire. And yet the end of the story was there all along, written in his name: Will-B, trapped in the future progressive tense, *an ongoing continuous action that would be occurring in the future.* A future that never arrives, because the future doesn't exist.

I had but one question for God: *What the f*ck?*

God didn't answer me. So I did the only ritual I knew to regain power, draw meaning from meaninglessness, feel whole and authoritative and divine. I would love to report that I strutted out of the bedroom and sat down at the kitchen table, full of purpose to wield my pen, but instead, I walked somberly and full of sorrow, feeling thrown, wearing a long T-shirt and no pants. I crossed the creaking floorboards into the dim dining room. I climbed up the wooden ladder to the attic. My navy blue meditation cushion was positioned under a skylight. I knelt down before it.

I opened my arms with nothing inside of them, ceremoniously handing the rest of my story over to the better care of God. Not because I was so pious and good, but because I wanted to be free. Then I climbed down the ladder and switched on the lamp.

FIFTY-SIX DAYS LATER, MY HAIR IS half-up in a beehive, a white veil covers my face. I am in the passenger's seat of a red 1975 Cadillac. I can't see the gathering of friends and family below because the road ahead is winding, but Mike is standing at the end. The cruise ship leaves tomorrow. Priestess school begins in one month. And I'm sitting on top of a mountain with a lifetime behind me, angling my face toward the sun, watching it flash through the veil.

ACKNOWLEDGMENTS

The line between "life" and "book" became all too fluid throughout the writing of this book. So I thank everyone I have ever met.

Nathaniel Jacks, for sending me an email that I was ninety percent sure was a scam because you and Inkwell Management seemed too good to be true. Thank you for believing in this book when it was just five pages long, for waiting five years for the full-blown manuscript, and for finding the perfect home with my dream publisher, Harper-One, and the consummate editor, Julia Pastore. Thank you Julia for being miraculously on point, every time, and for the brilliant insights that helped to shape this story. Jessie Dolch: genius copyeditor and writers' savior. Many thanks to the excellent team at HarperCollins: Eva Avery, Lisa Zuniga, and Victor Hendrickson. Nicole Caputo, natural born artist and pal, for the dazzling cover art, right up to the snakehead.

Gratitude to the following people whose guidance and suggestions, no matter how brief or long ago, pushed me forward: Mrs. Shrader, David Youngblood, Tony Thompson, Jeremy Jones, Greg Bottoms, Lisa Schnell, Lynne Greely, Patricia O'Toole, Leslie Sharpe, Kelly McMasters, Mary Karr, Lauren Slater, The Rev. Dr. Christian Brocato, and Marianne Williamson. Thanks to Samuel Freedman for teaching me about the business of writing a book. Susan Shapiro, literary rainmaker, my Jewish mother in New York.

Aspen Baker and Exhale champions Kate Hindman, Mayah Frank, Natalia Koss-Vallejo, Ronak Dave, Danielle Thomas, Thaler Pekar, Rich Snowden, and Sabrina Hersi Issa.

Chloe Caldwell, Josh Greenman, Daniel Jones, Leah Odze Epstein, HuffPost Live, Angie Aker, Jamil Smith, Melissa Harris Perry, Lizz Winstead, Sarah Silverman, Leigh Stein, and AWP for allowing me to share elements of this book with audiences.

Writers and friends who pruned drafts. Liza Monroy: bless you, woman. Elizabeth Greenwood, Deborah Jian Lee, Meaghan Winter, Meghan Finn, Abigail Rasminsky, Kelsey Motes-Connor, Gila Lyons, Melynda Fuller, Brian Spitulnik, Emily Herzlin, David Zax. Columbia and Sue Shapiro workshoppers. Freedman book seminar survivors. Anna Raskind, Ana Carano, and John Kelly, beautiful minds who contributed to research.

Friends: Travis, Anne, Terry, Bug, Miss Jordan, Mr. Carlos, Alex Hancock, Amanda Lockaby, Allison Faulconer, Krissy Ruddy, Kirsti McCracken, Karbaby, Marley Marosy, Jeannette Heindel, Jeanne Heaton, Mira Ptacin, Nadyia Brock, Mickey Svetich, Noland Chambliss, Jennifer Miller, Jason Feifer, Randi and Seth Rothschild, Terry Pierce, Harvest Henderson, Scott Wayne Indiana, Sara Faye Green, Kate Chapman.

To the women in the secret club: you are my grace.

To my sibs in the abortion club: you are my medicine.

To every stranger who emailed me or passed me an anonymous note of encouragement to keep writing this book through the years: your words showed up right on time.

Thank you, Binders.

From the depths of my heart, thank you to each and every person depicted in these pages—S.G., friends, family, and exes, priests, ministers, rabbis, therapists, scholars, and all others.

Thanks to friends and colleagues at Columbia and Harvard Divinity School. Thank you, Starbucks, Darwin's, the Hungarian Pastry Shop, Grounded, Butler Library, and Monika's Café Bar for allowing me to spend hours writing in your facilities—and to the banker at Capital One/Peet's Coffee & Tea, who *just now* handed me two coupons for free coffee, while I was typing this sentence. Evidence that you get what you're grateful for—sometimes instantly! Thank you Nicole Wallack, Sassons, Joshua Howes, Lindvalls, Christina Rumpf, for friendship and employment. Students at Columbia and Globe. Thank you to the great state of Kentucky.

Immense appreciation for the texts and truth-seekers whose words impacted this book: Bill Wilson, A Course in Miracles, Oprah, Michael Bernard Beckwith, Clarissa Pinkola Estes, Caroline Myss, and Iyanla Vanzant.

Joda, my trusted guide. This book could not exist without her.

Thanks to my whole family for being onboard with this book.

Thanks to my mother-in-law, who stocked her cupboard with my favorite foods and then handed me the keys to her empty apartment. Rock-and-roll aunts on all sides fed me food, art, and boundless support. Uncles. Cousins for their words of encouragement. Thanks to my grandparents for teaching me everything I know about exchanging ideas with people on opposite ends of the political spectrum, without trying to change anybody's mind. Thank you, T.R.U. for the spot-on professional advice and patient golf instruction. My brother is the funniest person on the planet. I lived for his phone calls (and 1930s southern accent) while I cranked out this volume. Thanks to my sister-in-law for her friendship and title votes. Thanks to my stepbrother.

Thanks to my dad for the countless hours on the phone and for titling Chapter Twenty "Spiritually Blonde" and for passing down an appreciation of "the strange and unusual"—which, no doubt, drew me into the spiritual adventure that develops in these pages.

Infinite gratitude to my mother whose contributions can't be quantified. Thanks for talking about this book without euphemism. Thanks for believing. Thanks to my stepfather for always weighing my suitcases on a bathroom scale before my flight. (Only books!)

Mike Murphy: all my love.

Thank you, God.

NOTES

Introduction: Email to My New Friend from the Internet

2 one in three American women . . . "Induced Abortion in the United States." Guttmacher Institute. May 2016. https://www.guttmacher.org/fact-sheet /induced-abortion-united-states.

Chapter 1: Hell

15 the Bush Administration allocated . . . "Chart of Total Federal Spending on Abstinence-Only-Until-Marriage Programs." SIECUS, Sexuality Information Counsel of the United States. October 19, 2011. http://www.siecus .org/index.cfm?fuseaction=document.showDocumentByID&DocumentID =72&varuniqueuserid=03652970735.

15 passing an unwrapped York Peppermint Pattie around the room . . . Alana Semuels, "Sex Education Stumbles in Mississippi." *Los Angeles Times,* April 2, 2014. http://www.latimes.com/nation/la-na-ms-teen-pregnancy-20140403 -story.html.

15 I had no idea . . . "International Abortion." Guttmacher Institute. http://www .guttmacher.org/media/presskits/abortion-WW/statsandfacts.html.

15 upward of fifty million abortions . . . "Induced Abortion Worldwide." Guttmacher Institute. 2016. https://www.guttmacher.org/fact-sheet/facts-induced -abortion-worldwide. More specifically, between 1990 and 1994, an estimated fifty million abortions occurred worldwide each year; between 2010 and 2014, this number had increased to an estimated fifty-six million per year, eighty-eight percent of which occurred in developing countries, where "an estimated 225 million women have an unmet need for modern contraceptives." By contrast, the abortion rate in developed countries dropped from twelve million to six million per year. Please visit the Guttmacher Institute webpage, listed above, to learn more about abortion rates around the globe and the circumstances and conditions surrounding people who find themselves in a position to terminate a pregnancy.

15 one in three American women . . . "Induced Abortion in the United States." Guttmacher Institute. May 2016. https://www.guttmacher.org/fact-sheet /induced-abortion-united-states.

24 I'd recently devoured Erica Jong's *Fear of Flying* . . . *Fear of Flying,* by Erica Jong. (New American Library, 2003), 17–18, 21.

Chapter 2: The End of April

35 There are 143 million orphans . . . "Children on the Brink 2004: A Joint Report of New Orphan Estimates and a Framework for Action." UNAIDS, UNICEF, and USAID. July 2004. http://www.unicef.org/publications/files/cob_layout6 -013.pdf.

35 Five hundred and eight thousand children . . . "Trends in Foster Care and Adoption: FFY 2002–FFY 2013." U.S. Department of Health and Human Services, Administration for Children and Families. Administration on Children, Youth and Families, Children's Bureau. https://www.acf.hhs.gov/sites/default /files/cb/trends_fostercare_adoption2013.pdf. By the end of the federal year 2004, the year this chapter took place, 508,000 children were in foster care in the U.S.; by the end of federal year 2013, 402,000 children were in foster care in the U.S. Please follow the link listed above to see a detailed chart.

36 According to antiabortion websites . . . "Abortion Information." 1st Way Life Center. http://www.1stwaylifecenter.com/abortion-information/.
Coleman, Priscilla. "Abortion Mental Health Research: Update and Quality of Evidence." *Association for Interdisciplinary Research in Values and Social Change Research Bulletin* 20, no. 2 (Spring 2008).
"Is Abortion Safe?" National Right to Life. http://www.nrlc.org/abortion /medicalfacts/safety/.

36 all symptoms of "postabortion syndrome" . . . "Are You Suffering from Post-Abortion Stress?" After Abortion. November 23, 1999. http://afterabortion .org/1999/are-you-suffering-from-post-abortion-stress/. Also see Theresa Burke's *Forbidden Grief: The Unspoken Pain of Abortion* (entire book).

36 pro-life psychologist named Vincent Rue . . . "Constitutional Amendments Relating to Abortion: hearings before the Subcommittee on the Constitution of the Committee on the Judiciary, United States Senate, Ninety-seventh Congress, first session, on S.J. Res. 17, S.J. Res. 18, S.J. Res. 19, and S.J. Res. 110 . . . October 5, 14, 19, November 4, 5, 12, 16, December 7, and 16, 1981." (1983), 329–339. See the testimony of Vincent Rue. To read the original transcript, please visit: https:// babel.hathitrust.org/cgi/pt?id=purl.32754062033141;view=1up;seq=343.

36 U.S. Surgeon General C. Everett Koop examined . . . "The C. Everett Koop Papers: Reproduction and Family Health." Profiles in Science: National Library of Science. https://profiles.nlm.nih.gov/ps/retrieve/Narrative/QQ/p-nid/88.

36 While the news media portrayed the physician . . . Following his initial report to the White House, Koop addressed the House Committee on Government Operations, The Subcommittee on Human Resources and Intergovernmental Relations, dated March 16, 1989, to elaborate on his conclusions and to correct the skewed and reductive media portrayal of his findings in a statement available online at: https://profiles.nlm.nih.gov/ps/access/QQBBQZ.pdf.

36 I have concluded in my review . . . "The Koop 'Non-Report,'" a letter from Koop to President Reagan dated January 9, 1989, is available to read online at Priests for Life. http://www.priestsforlife.org/postabortion/89-01-09koop.htm. Koop's letter also appears in *Abortion, Medicine, and the Law,* by J. Douglas Butler and David F. Walbert. (Fideli Publishing Inc.; Sixth Edition, 2011).

36 In 1989, the American Psychological Association . . . "Report of the APA Task Force on Mental Health and Abortion," by Brenda Major, Mark Appelbaum, Linda Beckman, Mary Ann Dutton, Nancy Felipe Russo, and Carolyn West. (American Psychological Association, Task Force on Mental Health and Abortion, 2008) 5. To read about the APA's 1989 report as well as its newer examination of scientific research conducted in 2008, please visit: http://www.apa.org/pi/women/programs/abortion/mental-health.pdf.

37 According to some of the most reputable reproductive health organizations . . . "Thinking about Abortion?" Planned Parenthood. https://www.plannedparenthood.org/learn/pregnancy/pregnant-now-what/thinking-about-abortion. "Abortion Facts," by Rene Almeling and Laureen Tews. National Abortion Federation. 1999. http://prochoice.org/education-and-advocacy/about-abortion/abortion-facts/.

Chapter 3: Crazy Love

51 If you want to understand any woman . . . *The Red Tent,* by Anita Diamant (Picador, 1997), 1.

52 Until you are the woman on the bricks . . . *Red Tent,* 168.

Chapter 4: The Bathroom Is My Prayer Temple

66 "craving for alcohol" . . . "Carl G. Jung's Letter to Bill Wilson," by Carl G. Jung. January 30, 1961. In A.A. History. http://www.barefootsworld.net/jungletter.html.

Chapter 5: One of Those Postabortion Meltdowns in Which I Question My Place in the Afterlife

80 In a study titled "Abortion as Stigma" . . . "Abortion as Stigma: Cognitive and Emotional Implications of Concealment," by Brenda Major and Richard H. Gramzow. *Journal of Personality and Social Psychology* 77, no. 4 (1999) 741, 742.

Chapter 6: "Rock-Bottom Loser Entertaining Offers from Several Religions"

91 find out what I'm thinking . . . "Why I write," by Joan Didion. The *New York Times Magazine* 5 (1976).

94 "She loved him so much it would kill her . . ." . . . *The Book of Laughter and Forgetting,* by Milan Kundera. (Harper Perennial, 1996), 202.

96 In a book titled . . . *Women of Wisdom,* by Tsultrim Allione (Routledge and Kegan Paul, 1984), 131.

97 An eighteenth-century nun named Orgyan Chokyi . . . *Himalayan Hermitess: The*

Life of a Tibetan Buddhist Nun, by Kurtis R. Schaeffer. (Oxford University Press, 2004), 46–49, 91, 143.

97 As the story goes . . . *When a Woman Becomes a Religious Dynasty,* by Hildegard Diemberger and Marilyn Strathern. Reprint ed. (Columbia University Press, 2014), 59.

99 the front page of the *New York Times* read . . . "Abortion Doctor Shot to Death in Kansas Church," by Joe Stumpe and Monica Davey. *New York Times,* May 31, 2009. http://www.nytimes.com/2009/06/01/us/01tiller.html ?pagewanted=all.

101 Buddhism began when a man who had everything . . . *The World's Religions: Our Great Wisdom Traditions,* by Huston Smith. (HarperSanFrancisco, 1991), 84–86.

103 Wikipedia page for 'hysteria' . . . "Hysteria." Wikipedia. https://en.wikipedia .org/wiki/Hysteria.

104 I found three ministrations . . . *Liquid Life: Abortion and Buddhism in Japan,* by William LaFleur. (Princeton University Press, 1992), 22–24.

105 the word *mizuko* means . . . *Liquid Life,* 16.

105 In Buddhism, we continually grow into our humanness . . . For information in this paragraph, see *Liquid Life,* 34–35, 39–41, 24, 26.

105 Japanese women created . . . *Liquid Life,* 126–27.

105 Evidence suggests that . . . *Liquid Life,* 126–27.

105 Japan had virtually no public debate . . . *Liquid Life,* 129.

105 There was a brief kerfuffle . . . *Abortion Before Birth Control: The Politics of Reproduction in Postwar Japan,* by Tiana Norgren. (Princeton University Press, 2001), 23.

105 *mabiki*—the Japanese word for thinning or pruning . . . *Liquid Life,* 99–100.

105 The government . . . distributed tablets . . . *Liquid Life,* 123, 128.

105 Women continued to end . . . *Liquid Life,* 123, 129.

107 Abortion has been practiced in India . . . "Re: Looking for an Indian Abortion Ritual," by Douglas Brooks. E-mail message to the author. August 25, 2010.

107 Though I did find a relevant quotation . . . *Hymns of the Atharva-Veda,* trans. Maurice Bloomfield. *The Sacred Books of the East,* Vol. XLII, ed. F. Max Müller (Clarendon, 1897), 165.

107 each school of Islam . . . *Islamic Ethics of Life: Abortion, War, and Euthanasia,* by Marion Holmes Katz, ed. Jonathan E. Brockopp. (University of South Carolina Press, 2003), 31.
Please read below for more information on the schools of Islam, with citations. All four schools of Sunni Islam thought—Maliki, Hanafi, Shafi'i, and Hanbali Schools—agree that abortion is forbidden after "ensoulment," or "the inbreathing of the spirit," which is believed to occur 120 days after conception. Before 120 days, there is no consensus among schools or, at times, even within them. Katz, *Islamic Ethics of Life,* 30.
The Maliki School strictly forbids abortion, some scholars describing it as "killing the soul," though it is permitted up to forty days under certain circumstances (mine would still be considered criminal).

"Controversies and Considerations regarding the Termination of Pregnancy for Foetal Anomalies in Islam," Abdulrahman Al-Matary and Jaffar Ali. *BMC Medical Ethics* 15, no. 1 (February 05, 2014): 652–57. http://www.ncbi.nlm.nih .gov/pmc/articles/PMC3943453/.

Islamic Ethics of Life: Abortion, War, and Euthanasia, by Donna Lee Bowen, ed. Jonathan E. Brockopp. (University of South Carolina Press, 2003), 78.

The Shafi'i School of thought is diverse, allowing abortion up to 120 days, forty-two days, or not at all.

Katz, *Islamic Ethics of Life,* 31.

The Hanbali School says up to forty days or until ensoulment.

Katz, *Islamic Ethics of Life,* 31.

The Hanafi School, on the other hand, regards terminations as permissible up to 120 days, though in some sects, the limit is set at forty days or determined by the circumstances of the pregnancy.

Katz, *Islamic Ethics of Life,* 31.

The Zahiri School forbids abortion, altogether, though does not consider it "killing."

Bowen, Katz, *Islamic Ethics of Life,* 78.

107 One set of instructions . . . "Abortion Fills Me With Remorse: How to Repent?" Islam Awareness. August 25, 2002. http://www.islamawareness.net/Family Planning/Abortion/abo_fatwa004.html.

Chapter 7: My Apology

114 statue of a man named Shinran Shonin . . . "F.Y.I.: Buddhist Bronze," by Ed Boland Jr. *New York Times,* November 3, 2002. http://www.nytimes.com /2002/11/03/nyregion/fyi-694762.html.

114 Buddha comes to earth . . . "Amida Buddha Is Everywhere," by Rev. Senpai Lewis-Bastias. BFF Podcasts. August 25, 2013. http://nelson.machighway .com/~bffnet/bffct/.

115 Inside the Buddhist church, I would . . . "Amida Buddha." 45, 127.

115 Bodhisattvas are gods and goddesses . . . "Amida Buddha." 46.

115 Their pre-Buddha status allows them . . . "Amida Buddha." 46.

115 The bodhisattva Jizo is said to understand . . . "Amida Buddha." 128.

115 He blesses future children. He blesses crossroads . . . "Amida Buddha." 49, 128–131.

115 He'd steer the little one . . . "Amida Buddha." 47–48, 128.

115 In certain sects of Buddhism . . . "Amida Buddha." 128.

115 Jizo corrects a water baby's karma . . . "Amida Buddha." 128.

115 dedicated solely to *mizuko kuyo* . . . "Amida Buddha." 5–10, 148, 153.

115 Japanese to pay respects to Jizos regularly . . . "Amida Buddha." 158–159.

115 In Japan, writes memoirist Marie . . . *Where the Dead Pause, and the Japanese Say Goodbye,* by Marie Mutsuki Mockett. (W. W. Norton, 2015), 201.

116 In the seventeenth century . . . *Liquid Life: Abortion and Buddhism in Japan,* 50–51, 113, 126–27.

116 Then she could meet . . . *Liquid Life,* 126–127, 148.

118 One purpose of the *mizuko kuyo* ritual . . . *Liquid Life,* 146–47.

Chapter 8: Suspicious Minds

Note: Four years after the retreat, I let Theresa Burke, "Linda," "Deacon Vince," "Corey," and "Don" know about my experience at Rachel's Vineyard and told them about this book. I also conducted follow-up interviews with "Amy," Steve, and "Tessa" and omitted the stories of anyone who did not return my emails.

Deacon Vince said, "I'll give this book to everyone I know! And I'll tell 'em, read this book before you do anything stupid!"

132 I was deeply disappointed . . . She was a student . . . See *The Gospel of Mary of Magdala: Jesus and the First Woman Apostle,* by Karen L. King. (Polebridge Press, 2003), 4–5.

132 raked through the mind . . . *The Mary Magdalene Cover-up. The Sources behind the Myth,* by Esther de Boer. (T&T Clark, 2007), 162–169, 172–181.

For more on the Magdalene Laundries, see *Origins of the Magdalene Laundries: An Analytical History,* by Rebecca Lea McCarthy. (McFarland & Company Publishers, 2010).

133 In 1994, a Roman Catholic psychologist . . . "What Is Rachel's Vineyard?" Rachel's Vineyard, *About Us.* 2016. http://www.rachelsvineyard.org/aboutus /index.aspx.

133 In a YouTube video, Burke explained . . . *Pro-Life Magazine* Interview with Dr. Theresa Burke of Rachel's Vineyard. YouTube, 2013. https://www.youtube .com/watch?v=yMUh8IfZZRw.

134 "better to marry than to burn" . . . *The Holy Bible, King James Version.* (American Bible Society, 1999), 1 Corinthians 7:9.

135 "Since the first century the Church . . . "Catechism of the Catholic Church," Part Three, "Life in Christ," 2271. http://www.vatican.va/archive/ccc_css /archive/catechism/p3s2c2a5.htm.

135 In 1869, Pope Pius IX had ruled . . . *Encyclopedia of Catholicism,* by Frank K. Flinn. (Facts on File, 2007), 3–4.

137 I studied the nameplate: Immaculate Conception . . . *Catechism of the Catholic Church.* 2nd ed. (Vatican City: Libreria Editrice Vaticana, 1994.) Part 1, Section 2, Chapter 2, Article 3, Paragraph 2, II, 490–493. http://www.vatican.va /archive/ccc_css/archive/catechism/p122a3p2.htm.

141 when she was sixteen, she told me . . . Phone interview with Linda, March 2014.

141 Tactics included praying loudly . . . For further reading on the effects of clinic protesters, please see: "6 Women on Their Terrifying, Infuriating Encounters With Abortion Clinic Protesters," by Liz Welch. *Cosmopolitan,* February 21, 2014. http://www.cosmopolitan.com/politics/news/a5669/abortion -clinic-protesters/.

See also: Chapter 10, "Thirty Second of Grief."

See also: *Dispatches from The Abortion Wars: The Costs of Fanaticism to Doctors, Patients, and The Rest of Us* by Carole Joffe. (Beacon Press, 2010).

141 Volunteers in orange or yellow vests . . . For further reading about clinic escorts, including an army veteran who volunteers to protect people entering clinics named Paul Valette, please see: "Meet The People Who Provide Protection At Abortion Clinics," by Alex Zielinski. *ThinkProgress,* December 9, 2015. http://thinkprogress.org/health/2015/12/09/3729440/clinic-escort-stories/. See also: "They Call Me 'The Devil': What It's Like To Be An Escort At Mississippi's Last Remaining Abortion Clinic" by Lori Gregory-Garrott. *Slate,* July 23, 2013. NOTE: Disturbing video, not for everyone. http://www.slate .com/articles/double_x/doublex/2013/07/mississippi_s_last_abortion_ clinic_what_it_s_like_to_be_an_escort_on_the.html.

For anyone who has ever felt hurt by clinic protesters, here is a cathartic video: in London, a pregnant woman who works for a children's charity erupts in moral outrage at a protester filming women entering an abortion clinic. (NOTE: Background image may be disturbing to some.) "Pregnant woman blasts anti-abortion protesters outside a clinic in London." https://www.you-tube.com/watch?v=XMy-V1TIoHI.

144 The narrator, a woman wearing shoulder pads that extended from coast to coast . . . "Abortion & Informed Consent—American Women Don't Need A Lecture?," by Theresa Karminski Burke, Ph.D. Rachel's Vineyard Ministries. http://www.rachelsvineyard.org/PDF/Articles/Abortion%20and%20 Informed%20Consent%20-%20Theresa%20Burke.pdf.

A helpful resource to understand the conflicting studies about abortion and breast cancer: "Is Abortion Linked to Breast Cancer?" American Cancer Society. June 19, 2014. http://www.cancer.org/cancer/breastcancer/moreinformation /is-abortion-linked-to-breast-cancer. This review is reasonably digestible and makes no bones about the challenges of gathering accurate information about abortion and breast cancer in a social climate in which researchers and study participants alike might feel passionately about abortion—either pro or anti. In "case-control studies," researchers face a problem called "recall bias." Study participants who are living with the disease under consideration (breast cancer, in this case) are more likely to try hard to remember aspects of their past that could have contributed to developing the disease. They are also more likely to disclose private and sometimes embarrassing facts about themselves. The "control" set of study participants (those without breast cancer, in this case) might not feel as motivated to disclose private facts about themselves, such as a past abortion. A "cohort study" gathers information on study participants as they move through their lives. This is supposed to be a more accurate method, though people still might not feel comfortable disclosing an abortion.

I have met women who never disclose their abortions on medical forms; who paid in cash to keep it off their medical records; who use euphemisms such as "forced miscarriage"; who forgot that they had one in the first place. The

American Cancer Society concludes that, "At this time, the scientific evidence does not support the notion that abortion of any kind raises the risk of breast cancer or any other type of cancer." (Full disclosure: the ACS does not have a spotless conflict-of-interest record.) Theresa Burke, the founder of Rachel's Vineyard, has argued that studies linking abortion and breast cancer have been suppressed. If there is any truth to Burke's assertion, it is obvious why such studies would be suppressed. Any negative information associated with abortion stokes the anti-abortion movement's efforts to hinder access to abortion rights, even though the evidence wouldn't be compelling. Some people would have an abortion even if an unbiased study showed that it might cause breast cancer. Before 1973, Americans used household appliances to induce abortion, even though they knew they might die of septic shock. The threat of physical problems after an abortion has never stopped people from procuring them, but the threat of abortion rights has consistently stopped professionals and study participants from being able to produce balanced results.

It is my contention that as long as research about abortion is motivated by even a subtle political agenda, producing a study with universal appeal will be virtually impossible.

144 But even "scientific studies" validated by the secular establishment could be biased . . . Here is a funny and entertaining critique of "scientific studies," subtle bias, and "bullshit masquerading as science": "Scientific Studies: Last Week Tonight with John Oliver" (HBO). May 8, 2016. https://www.youtube.com/watch?v=0Rnq1NpHdmw.

155 The Church is aware of the many factors . . . "Evangelium Vitae," by Pope John Paul II. 1995. http://w2.vatican.va/content/john-paul-ii/en/encyclicals/documents/hf_jp-ii_enc_25031995_evangelium-vitae.html.

Chapter 10: Thirty Seconds of Grief

168 two well-documented suicides of pregnant women . . . Two formerly pregnant ghosts: Kate Morgan and the woman from Room 3502: Stacey V. Levinson, "Coronado Is Haunted," *San Diego Reader,* February 8, 2013. http://www.sandiegoreader.com/news/2013/feb/08/travel-haunted-coronado-california/. Also, Diane Hunter, "The Ghost of the Del: The Secret of Room 3502," *Orange Coast: The Magazine of Orange County,* October 1990, available on Google Books. Also, Walter Bissell, "Haunted Hotel Del Coronado," *Angels & Ghosts,* http://www.angelsghosts.com/hotel_del_coronado_famous_haunted_place_story.

170 People had been having abortions since ancient times . . . "Abortion and Medicine: A Sociopolitical History," by Carole Joffe. February 13, 2009. http://media.wiley.com/product_data/excerpt/62/14051769/1405176962.pdf.

170 Plato and Aristotle supported it . . . "Women and Family in Athenian Law," by K. Kapparis. Center for Hellenic Studies. Harvard University. http://chs.harvard.edu/CHS/article/display/1190.

170 A textbook containing a Persian doctor's . . . "Abortion and Medicine."

171 To my surprise, there was a time . . . *Women and Health in America: Historical Readings,* by Judith Walzer Leavitt. (University of Wisconsin Press, 1999), 270.

171 Black women in slavery exchanged stories . . . "Whitewashing Reproductive Rights: How Black Activists Get Erased," by Renee Bracey Sherman. *Salon,* February 24, 2014. http://www.salon.com/2014/02/25/whitewashing _reproductive_rights_how_black_activists_get_erased/.

171 Then, the American Medical Association advocated . . . *Women and Health in America,* 270.

171 During the Victorian Age in the United States and England . . . Library of Congress. Serial and Government Publications Division. "Advertisements." http:// memory.loc.gov/ammem/awhhtml/awser2/advertisement.html.

171 Women used branded medicines . . . *Abortion Care,* by Sam Rowlands. (Cambridge University Press, 2014), 62.

171 alias for Ann Trow Lohman . . . *The Crimes of Womanhood: Defining Femininity in a Court of Law,* by Cheree A. Carlson. (University of Illinois Press, 2009), 112.

171 famous nineteenth-century abortionist who lived in a swanky apartment on Fifth Avenue . . . "MADAME RESTELL: Lies Mouldering in Her Grave, But Her Heirs Are Marching On DID SHE MURDER HER HUSBAND? Upon the Solution of This Question Depends the Possession of Ill-Gotten Wealth A STRANGE DEATH-BED SCENE," *National Police Gazette,* May 15, 1880, 36th ed., sec. 138.

171 had an impressive criminal record . . . *The Crimes of Womanhood: Defining Femininity in a Court of Law,* by Cheree A. Carlson. (University of Illinois Press, 2009), 117–122.

171 From 1938 to the 1950s, the Detroit-based physician . . . "Whitewashing Reproductive Rights."

171 Women also had abortions blindfolded . . . "Blindfolded, I Had an Abortion in 1970," by Jean Panella. *Ms. Magazine,* January 22, 2016. http://msmagazine. com/blog/2016/01/22/blindfolded-i-had-an-abortion-in-1970/; "Will We Return to the Trauma of Blindfolded Abortions?," by Clark Morphew. *Orlando Sentinel,* March 10, 2001. http://articles.orlandosentinel.com/2001-03-10 /lifestyle/0103090470_1_abortions-young-women-wealthy-family; *When Abortion Was a Crime: Women, Medicine, and Law in the United States, 1867–1973,* by Leslie J. Reagan. (University of California Press, 1997), 243.

171 acid, cottonseed oil, quinine and chloroquine . . . black market herbs . . . a bicycle spoke, a coat hanger, a knitting needle . . . or a lump of sugar: "Unsafe Abortion: The Preventable Pandemic," by David A. Grimes, Janie Benson, Susheela Singh, Mariana Romero, Bela Ganatra, Friday E. Okonofua, and Iqbal H. Shah. *The Lancet* 368, no. 9550 (2006): 1911. http://www.thelancet.com /journals/lancet/article/PIIS0140673606694816/abstract.

171 turpentine, bleach . . . "Unsafe Abortion: Unnecessary Maternal Mortality," by Lisa B. Haddad and Nawal M. Nour. *Reviews in Obstetrics and Gynecology* 2, no. 2 (Spring 2009): 123. http://www-ncbi-nlm-nih-gov.ezp-prod1.hul.harvard.edu /pmc/articles/PMC2709326/.

171 pounding the belly with a pestle . . . "Thousand-year-old depictions of massage abortion," by Malcolm Potts, Maura Graff, and Judy Taing. *Journal of Family Planning and Reproductive Health Care* 33, no. 4 (2007): 233–234. http://bixby .berkeley.edu/wp-content/uploads/2015/03/Thousand-year-old-depictions -of-massage-abortion.pdf.

171 leeches . . . "Leeches, Lye and Spanish Fly," by Kate Manning. *New York Times,* January 21, 2013. http://www.nytimes.com/2013/01/22/opinion/leeches-lye -and-spanish-fly.html?_r=0.

172 Next I read Ava's story . . . Ava's mother's story and Ava's story are told in *Peace After Abortion,* by Ava Torre-Bueno. 2nd ed. (Pimpernel, 1997), 4–5. Also interviews conducted by the author, June 2010 and November 2012.

172 It was fairly common for doctors . . . *Our Bodies, Ourselves for the New Century,* by Boston Women's Health Book Collective. (Touchstone, 1998), 408.

172 The number of unlawful abortions before 1973 . . . "Lessons from Before Roe: Will Past Be Prologue?," by Rachel Benson Gold, Guttmacher Institute, Guttmacher Policy Review, March 1, 2003. http://www.guttmacher.org/pubs/tgr /06/1/gr060108.html.

172 compared with today's rate of . . . "Induced Abortion in the United States." Guttmacher Institute, March 2016. http://www.guttmacher.org/pubs/tgr/06/1 /gr060108.html.

172 An estimated five thousand women died of unsafe . . . "The Safety of Legal Abortion and the Hazards of Illegal Abortion." NARAL Pro-Choice America. http://www.prochoiceamerica.org/media/fact-sheets/abortion-distorting -science-safety-legal-abortion.pdf.

175 According to Theresa Burke . . . "Dr. Theresa Burke Interviewed by *Pro-Life Magazine.*" Interview. *Pro-Life Magazine,* December 31, 2013. 12:20–12:50. https://www.youtube.com/watch?v=lrWUR0sITYY.

177 Egyptian culture . . . Balinese . . . "Bereavement and Loss in Two Muslim Communities: Egypt and Bali Compared," by Wikan U. *Soc Sci Med.* 1988; 27(5): 451–60. Abstract at http://www.ncbi.nlm.nih.gov/pubmed/3227353.

177 During the Victorian Age, women dressed . . . "Victorian Mourning Etiquette." http://www.tchevalier.com/fallingangels/bckgrnd/mourning/.

178 In the Greco-Roman world . . . "Women's Tears in Ancient Roman Ritual," by Darja Šterbenc Erker, in *Tears in the Graeco-Roman World,* ed. Thorsten Fogen (Walter de Gruyter, 2009), 135–60.

179 complicated grief . . . "COMPLICATED GRIEF AND RELATED BEREAVEMENT ISSUES FOR DSM-5," by Katherine M. Shear. *Depression and Anxiety.* U.S. National Library of Medicine, February, 2011.

Chapter 11: How to Take Up Space

188 In *Waking the Tiger: Healing Trauma* . . . *Waking the Tiger: Healing Trauma: The Innate Capacity to Transform Overwhelming Experiences,* by Peter A. Levine. (North Atlantic Books, 1997), 61–2.

Chapter 12: Another Underground Movement

195 Backline was a phone counseling service . . . Backline. https://www.yourback line.org.

195 Exhale, an after-abortion talkline . . . Exhale. https://exhaleprovoice.org/after -abortion-talkline.

197 In "(Mis)understanding Abortion Regret," she reported . . . "(Mis)Understanding Abortion Regret," by Katrina Kimport. *Symbolic Interaction*, Vol. 3, Issue 2. 2012, 105.

197 phone counselors at two secular talklines supporting people after abortion . . . Ibid., 108.

198 About half of potential study participants . . . Ibid., 109.

204 Now, this Baker babe . . . Limbaugh quoted in *Pro-Voice: How to Keep Listening When the World Wants a Fight*, by Aspen Baker (Berrett-Koehler, 2015), 101–102.

204 More than five thousand abortion e-cards were sent . . . *Pro-Voice*, 104.

Chapter 14: Manifesto of the Three Billion Sluts

219 One million women in France have an abortion every year . . . "Manifesto343." Manifesto343. http://www.bibme.org/bibliographies/159890084?new=true.

220 Across the world, humans have had approximately three billion recorded abortions . . . "Induced Abortion Worldwide." Guttmacher Institute. 2016. https:// www.guttmacher.org/fact-sheet/facts-induced-abortion-worldwide. Annually, about fifty-six million abortions occur worldwide. At this rate—which shifts, year to year—it would take 53.6 years to reach three billion abortions.

225 I'm pregnant. I just found out. . . . "I'm Having an Abortion This Weekend," by Jenny Kutner. *Salon*, August 1, 2014. http://www.salon.com/2014/08/01 /im_having_an_abortion_this_weekend/.

226 If I used birth control and had sex . . . *Lizz Free or Die*, by Lizz Winstead. (Riverhead, 2012), 72.

226 I don't think the punishment . . . Renee Bracey Sherman interview with the author, June 17, 2015.

226 I didn't realize that if you're throwing up the Pill . . . "16 and Pregnant: No Easy Decision," MTV, 2009–2014. http://www.mtv.ca/shows/16-and-pregnant /video/extras/16-and-pregnant-no-easy-decision-special/1655243/0/4. Note: this web address changes often; if the link above does not work, please Google: "16 and Pregnant: No Easy Decision." (Be sure to include the quotation marks.)

226 I chose food over birth control . . . Katie Klabusich interview with the author, July 4, 2014.

226 A baby meant the destruction of everything . . . "Talking About My Abortion," by Molly Crabapple. *VICE*, August 5, 2013. http://www.vice.com/read /about-my-abortion.

226 I was broke, unmarried, restless . . . "Childless, With Regret and Advice: Don't Wait for the Perfect Picture," by Susan Shapiro. Motherload: Living

the Family Dynamic. *New York Times,* January 23, 2015. http://parenting
.blogs.nytimes.com/2015/01/23/childless-with-regret-and-advice-dont-wait
-for-the-perfect-picture/.

226 I had published three books by then . . . *Traveling Mercies: Some Thoughts On Faith,*
by Anne Lamott. (Pantheon, 1999), 48.

226 I'm on Accutane . . . *Unbreak My Heart: A Memoir,* by Toni Braxton. (Harper-
Collins, 2014), 177.

226 I was afraid [that my mother] would withdraw . . . *Her Choice to Heal: Finding Spiritual and Emotional Peace After Abortion,* by Sydna Masse. (David C. Cook, 2009), 37.

226 We're broke kids . . . "Meet The Girl Who's Crowdfunding Her Abortion," by
Troy Farah. *VICE,* September 5, 2014. http://www.vice.com/read/meet-the
-girl-whos-crowdfunding-her-abortion-905.

227 I didn't have the mental capacity . . . "The View" Fights over Abortion, You-
Tube, RandomClips2008, https://www.youtube.com/watch?v=4d_gumas_l4.

227 We're always the image of a black woman . . . Renee Bracey Sherman interview
with the author, June 17, 2015.

227 I wasn't ready . . . "Nicki Minaj Is Hip-Hop's Killer Diva: Inside Rolling Stone's
New Issue." *Rolling Stone,* December 30, 2014. http://www.rollingstone.com
/music/news/nicki-minaj-is-hip-hops-killer-diva-inside-rolling-stones-new
-issue-20141230.

227 We'd set up our kids to fail . . . "16 and Pregnant: No Easy Decision."

227 I've been without water . . . "16 and Pregnant: No Easy Decision."

227 Irregular heart structure, no brain development . . . "Un-bearing," by Mira
Ptacin. *Guernica,* March 1, 2012. https://www.guernicamag.com/features
/ptacin_3_1_12/.

227 Trisomy, a triple chromosome . . . *Bad Mother: A Chronicle of Maternal Crimes, Minor Calamities, and Occasional Moments of Grace,* by Ayelet Waldman. (Doubleday,
2009), 124.

227 I acknowledged it as a baby . . . "16 and Pregnant: No Easy Decision."

227 Pregnancy felt like a mixture . . . "Talking About My Abortion."

227 I love milk . . . Renee Bracey Sherman interview with the author, June 17, 2015.

227 I felt like somebody had invaded my uterus . . . Katie Klabusich interview with
the author, July 4, 2014.

227 I raged against my body . . . "Un-bearing."

227 I felt unattractive in an entirely new way . . . "Abortion, a Love Story," by
Gila Lyons. *Salon,* August 25, 2012. http://www.salon.com/2012/08/25
/abortion_a_love_story/.

227 I enjoyed being pregnant . . . Aspen Baker interview with the author, April 14,
2010.

228 If we do what you want to do . . . *Bad Mother,* 128.

228 Ayelet had once notoriously confessed . . . "Truly, Madly, Guiltily," by Ayelet
Waldman. *New York Times,* March 27, 2005. http://www.nytimes.com/2005
/03/27/fashion/truly-madly-guiltily.html.

228 Iman Ahmed, a devout Muslim . . . "A Muslimah's Story—I Chose to Have an Abortion," by Iman Ahmed. *altmuslim* (blog), *Part One,* June 7, 2013: http://www.patheos.com/blogs/altmuslim/2013/06/a-muslimahs-story-i -chose-to-have-an-abortion-part-one/. Part Two, June 10, 2013: http://www .patheos.com/blogs/altmuslim/2013/06/a-muslimahs-story-i-chose-to-have -an-abortion-part-two/.

228 Underneath it all . . . "Abortion, a Love Story."

228 The father was someone I had just met . . . *Traveling Mercies,* 48.

228 He had an eighth-grade education . . . Renee Bracey Sherman interview with the author, June 17, 2015.

228 I began to distance myself . . . *Her Choice to Heal,* 37.

228 I feel I chose to end my baby's life . . . *Bad Mother,* 131.

228 a Jewish embryo . . . "Abortion, a Love Story."

229 A river of blood the second day . . . "Abortion, a Love Story."

229 I was clearly far from . . . "A Muslimah's Story."

229 I promise, NO MORE SEX . . . *Lizz Free or Die,* 78.

229 I'd made a choice . . . *Unbreak My Heart,* 179.

229 The first thing I thought when I awoke . . . "I Couldn't Turn My Abortion into Art," by Lisa Selin Davis. *New York Times,* July 2, 2014. http://opinionator .blogs.nytimes.com/2014/07/02/i-couldnt-turn-my-abortion-into-art/.

229 I have mixed emotions right now . . . "16 and Pregnant: No Easy Decision."

229 I keep waiting for my prescribed grief . . . *How to Be a Woman,* by Caitlin Moran. (Harper Perennial, 2012), 276.

229 Most of my discomfort . . . "How Should an Abortion Be?," by Monica Heisey. *Gawker,* January 22, 2015. http://gawker.com/how-should-an-abortion-be-1680939464.

229 She shouldn't be afraid . . . *The Empathy Exams,* by Leslie Jamison. (Graywolf Press, 2014), 11.

229 Because I believed abortions . . . "Talking About My Abortion."

229 I wish that someone had alerted me . . . "I Couldn't Turn My Abortion into Art."

229 I would never recommend . . . "Coming Out on Abortion," The Opinion Pages, Room for Debate. *New York Times,* June 30, 2013. http://www.nytimes.com /roomfordebate/2013/06/30/coming-out-on-abortion.

230 I don't want a child . . . "Chelsea Handler on Rosie," YouTube, February 8, 2012. https://www.youtube.com/watch?v=v5YGXL0-g8M.

230 About motherhood, though . . . "I Couldn't Turn My Abortion into Art."

230 What seemed tragic was . . . "Childless, with Regret and Advice: Don't Wait for the Perfect Picture."

230 My abortion made me look at my life . . . Renee Bracey Sherman interview with the author, June 17, 2015.

230 I'm a man . . . "Guest Post: I'm a Man and I Had An Abortion." *The Belle Jar,* October 14, 2015. http://bellejar.ca/2015/10/14/guest-post-im-a-man-and-i -had-an-abortion/.

230 I had an abortion when I was seventeen, and I didn't . . . "Why I Started a Podcast About Abortion," by Robin Marty. *Cosmopolitan,* September 17, 2014. http://www.cosmopolitan.com/politics/interviews/a31137/abortion-diaries/.

230 I just want women and girls . . . "16 and Pregnant: No Easy Decision."

230 It saved my life to know . . . "Ayelet Waldman: Bad Mother," by Belinda Luscombe. *Time,* May 8, 2009. http://content.time.com/time/arts/article/0,8599 ,1896848,00.html.

Chapter 15: A Marginally Advanced Understanding of My Mother

237 Automatic writing is believed to have been . . . *Zohar: Annotated & Explained,* by Daniel C. Matt. (Skylight Paths, 2002).

Chapter 16: Wild Woman

246 Schiff told me (because books talk to me) that Jewish law . . . The word halakhah means to go, to walk . . . *Abortion in Judaism,* by Daniel Schiff. (Cambridge University Press, 2002), vii.

247 Schiff writes: "A competent rabbinic authority must be consulted . . ." . . . *Abortion in Judaism,* viii.

247 a feminist named Arlene Agus . . . "This month is for you: observing Rosh Hodesh as a woman's holiday," by Arlene Agus. *The Jewish Woman: New Perspectives.* (Schocken, 1976), 84–93.
      See also: "Feminist Recalls Festival's Comeback," by Jill Huber. *New Jersey Jewish News.* January 22, 2008. http://njjewishnews.com/njjn.com/012408 /moFeministRecalls.html.

248 the third most holy site in Jerusalem . . . "Holy Site Sparks Row between Israel and UN," Ana Carbajosa. *The Guardian.* October 29, 2010. https://www.the guardian.com/world/2010/oct/29/religious-site-israel-united-nations.

248 pioneering badass in Germany . . . "1935: World's First Female Rabbi Is Ordained, in Germany—This Day in Jewish History," by David B. Green. *Haaretz.* December 27, 2015. http://www.haaretz.com/israel-news/2.489/.premium-1 .693942.

248 the first female Reform rabbi . . . "Sally Jane Priesand," by Pamela S. Nadell. *Jewish Women: A Comprehensive Historical Encyclopedia.* March 1, 2009. Jewish Women's Archive. http://jwa.org/encyclopedia/article/priesand-sally-jane.

248 the first female Reconstructionist rabbi . . . Conservative Judaism wouldn't ordain . . . Orthodox Judaism does not ordain female rabbis . . . "Women in Judaism: A History of Women's Ordination as Rabbis," by Avi Hein. Jewish Virtual Library. http://www.jewishvirtuallibrary.org/jsource/Judaism/female rabbi.html.

249 When I congratulated Rayzel on penning the first Jewish abortion ritual in 1992 . . . Rabbi Pamela Frydman created a ritual specifically for cult survivors who have terminated pregnancies. Hers was actually the first unrecorded Jewish abortion ritual in America. For those interested in ritual for

cult survivors, Rabbi Frydman generously allowed its inclusion here:
"This ritual is for everyone who has had an abortion or is preparing to have one, for those became pregnant in a loving way or through force, trauma or tragedy. This was created as a religious ritual and can be used by anyone of any faith or no faith.

The ritual has four elements—candle, remembering, speaking with the soul, closing prayer.

Candle—Choose a candle you like that burns for a long time. Light the candle for yourself and the being who has come to grow in your womb. If you are Jewish, feel free to use a yahrzeit or shiva candle, or any other candle of your choice. Remembering—Take your time. Remember what happened that led you to make the decision, or be faced with the decision to not carry this being to term. Be gentle with yourself. If you are doing this ritual alone, feel free to express yourself in silence or talk out loud. If you are doing this ritual with others, ask for what you need from them that will help to remember and talk about your remembering.

The Soul—Talk with the soul. Tell the soul what you want the soul to know. Do you want to invite the soul to come back later, at a later time in your life? Or shall you invite the soul to find a new womb to bring the soul into the world? Do you want to ask for forgiveness or to say thank you?

Closing Prayer or Wish—Express this as a wish or a prayer, depending on your belief and what feels right. What do you wish for yourself? For the soul of the being that was or will be aborted? For your loved one(s)? For your abuser(s)? For others who may be involved? For Jewish practitioners: In addition to the prayer(s) or wish(es) that you choose for this ritual, also include Baruch Dayan HaEmet. Blessed is the Judge of Truth. These are words recited when we hear news of a death. Whether you have had an abortion recently or long ago or if you are about to have an abortion, in either case, these are appropriate words if you wish to recite them. Amen."

249 After Rayzel, the next recorded ritual . . . "Updated Manual for Rabbis Issued." *Los Angeles Times*. October 24, 1998. http://articles.latimes.com/1998/oct/24/local/me-35635.

249 In *Taking Up the Timbrel: The Challenge of Creating Ritual for Jewish Women Today* . . . *Taking up the Timbrel: The Challenge of Creating Ritual for Jewish Women Today* by Sylvia Rothschild and Sybil Sheridan. (SCM Press, 2000).

250 Before visitors submerge in the waters . . . . . . "FAQs." Mayyim Hayyim. http://www.mayyimhayyim.org/About/FAQs.

250 Mayyim Hayyim supports religious pluralism . . . . . . "FAQs." Mayyim Hayyim. http://www.mayyimhayyim.org/About/FAQs.

Chapter 19: Hardcore Feminist Texas Church Ladies

294 Halfway through my pregnancy . . . "'We Have No Choice': One Woman's Ordeal with Texas' New Sonogram Law," by Carolyn Jones. *Texas Ob-*

server, March 15, 2012. https://www.texasobserver.org/we-have-no-choice -one-womans-ordeal-with-texas-new-sonogram-law/.

295 Enforcing "ambulatory center standards" . . . For an update on the ruling, in which the Supreme Court struck down such standards, please visit: https:// www.supremecourt.gov/opinions/15pdf/15-274_p8k0.pdf.

295 Hospitals already admitted patients . . . "Safety of Abortion in the United States." ANSIRH: Advancing New Standards in Reproductive Health. December 2014. http://www.ansirh.org/sites/default/files/publications/files/safety brief12-14.pdf.

296 To mock the old-fashioned bill . . . "Perry's Special Session: A Cruel Summer for Abortion Rights," by Carolyn Jones. *Texas Observer*, June 14, 2013. http://www.texasobserver.org/perrys-special-session-a-cruel-summer-for -abortion-rights/. Activists in North Carolina used the same strategy: "North Carolina Women Don 1960s Garb to Protest 'Vintage' Bill That Threatens Birth Control Access," by Tara Culp-Ressler. *ThinkProgress*, May 15, 2013. http://thinkprogress.org/health/2013/05/15/2016881/north -carolina-birth-control-access-vintage/.

297 thousands of criminal activities . . . "NAF Violence and Disruption Statistics." National Abortion Federation, 2014. http://5aa1b2xfmfh2e2mk03kk8rsx .wpengine.netdna-cdn.com/wp-content/uploads/Stats_Table_2014.pdf.

297 In Nebraska in 1991 an arsonist . . . "Roe versus Reality: Abortion and Women's Health," by Alexi A. Wright and Ingrid T. Katz. *New England Journal of Medicine*, 355: 1–9, July 6, 2006. http://www.nejm.org/doi/full/10.1056 /NEJMp068083.

297 And the slaying of Dr. George Tiller . . . "Abortion Doctor Shot to Death in Kansas Church," by Joe Stumpe and Monica Davey. *New York Times*, May 31, 2009. http://www.nytimes.com/2009/06/01/us/01tiller.html?pagewanted=all.

297 All across the United States . . . In the ten years between 2001 and 2010, 205 restrictions had been imposed; in the three years between 2011 and 2013, 204 restrictions.

297 Over the course of two years, up to two hundred thousand . . . "Knowledge, Opinion, and Experience Related to Abortion Self-Induction in Texas," by D. Grossman, K. White, L. Fuentes, K. Hopkins, A. Stevenson, S. Yeatman, and J. E. Potter. Texas Policy Evaluation Project, November 14, 2015. https://utexas .app.box.com/KOESelfInductionResearchBrief.

297 A *New York Times* graph showed . . . "The Return of the D.I.Y. Abortion" by Seth Stephens-Davidowitz. *New York Times*, March 5, 2016. http://www.nytimes .com/2016/03/06/opinion/sunday/the-return-of-the-diy-abortion.html.

ABOUT THE AUTHOR

KASSI UNDERWOOD is a writer and a lecturer who grew up in Lexington, Kentucky. Her work has been published in the *New York Times*, *The Atlantic* online, *The Rumpus*, *Refinery29*, and *Guernica*, among others. She holds an MFA from Columbia University, where she taught on the faculty of the Undergraduate Writing Program. She has been a guest on MSNBC and HuffPost Live, profiled in the *New York Magazine* cover story, "My Abortion," alongside twenty-five other women, and a speaker at colleges and faith communities nationwide. Kassi lectures about personal transformation, addiction recovery, social justice, and the spirituality of abortion. She is a student at Harvard Divinity School and co-host of the podcast *Spiritually Blonde*.

Connect with Kassi online:

Visit: www.kassiunderwood.com

Follow on Twitter and Instagram: @kassiunderwood

Like the Facebook page: @kassiunderwood